W0090503

Physiotherapy in Pregnancy

Antenatal, Postnatal and Baby Care

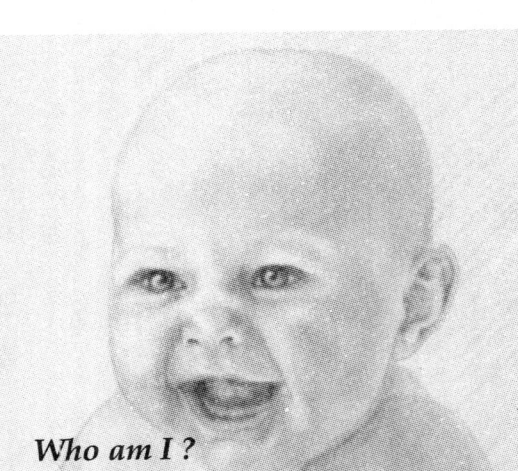

Who am I ?

I am the Seed of Life
I am the Product of Multiplication
I am the Origin of Creation
I am the Symbol of Love
I am the Light of Almighty
I am the Figure of Nature
Yes, I am One among U
I am the Miniature form of U
Aha ! I am the Glowing Gift of God
I am the Seed of Life !

Physiotherapy in Pregnancy

Antenatal, Postnatal and Baby Care

Malti Hiranandani
Assistant Professor

and

Vandana Balaji
Assistant Professor

Apollo College of Physiotherapy
Apollo Hospital
Hyderabad

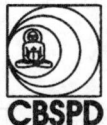

CBSPD

CBS Publishers & Distributors Pvt Ltd

New Delhi • Bengaluru • Chennai • Kochi • Kolkata • Mumbai
Hyderabad • Jharkhand • Nagpur • Patna • Pune • Uttarakhand

Disclaimer

Science and technology are constantly changing fields. New research and experience broaden the scope of information and knowledge. The authors have tried their best in giving information available to them while preparing the material for this book. Although all efforts have been made to ensure optimum accuracy of the material, yet it is quite possible some errors might have been left uncorrected. The publisher, the printer and the authors will not be held responsible for any inadvertent errors, omissions or inaccuracies.

Physiotheraphy in Pregnancy

ISBN: 978-81-239-1229-5

First Edition: 2005
Reprint: 2006, 2010, 2013, 2015, 2018, 2020, **2025**

Copyright © Authors and Publisher

All rights reserved. No part of this book may be reproduced or transmitted in any form or by any means, electronic or mechanical, including photocopying, recording, or any information storage and retrieval system without the permission, in writing, from the authors and the publisher.

Published by **Satish Kumar Jain** and produced by **Varun Jain** for

CBS Publishers & Distributors Pvt Ltd
4819/XI Prahlad Street, 24 Ansari Road, Daryaganj, New Delhi 110 002, India.
Ph: 011-23266838, 23289259   Website: www.cbspd.com
e-mail: delhi@cbspd.com

Corporate Office: 204 FIE, Industrial Area, Patparganj, Delhi 110 092
Ph: 011-4934 4934   Fax: 011-4934 4935
e-mail: publishing@cbspd.com; publicity@cbspd.com

Branches

- **Bengaluru:** Seema House 2975, 17th Cross, KR Road, Banasankari 2nd Stage, Bengaluru 560 070, Karnataka, India
  Ph: +91-80-26771678/79   Fax: +91-80-26771680   e-mail: bangalore@cbspd.com
- **Chennai:** 18/8B, Subbarayan Street, Shenoy Nagar, Chennai 600 030, Tamil Nadu, India
  Ph: +91-44-42032115, 26681266   e-mail: chennai@cbspd.com
- **Kochi:** 42/1325, 1326, Power House Road, Opp KSEB, Power House, Ernakulum Kochi 682 018, Kerala, India
  Ph: +91-484-4059061-65,67   Fax: +91-484-4059065   e-mail: kochi@cbspd.com
- **Kolkata:** 147. Hind Ceramics Compound, 1st Floor, Nilgunj Road, Belghoria, Kolkata-700056, West Bengal, India
  Ph: +033-25633055, 033-25633056   e-mail: kolkata@cbspd.com
- **Lucknow:** Basement, Khushnuma Complex, 7 Meerabai Marg (Behind Jawahar Bhawan), Lucknow-226001, UP, India
  Ph: +0522-4000032   e-mail: tiwari.lucknow@cbspd.com
- **Mumbai:** PWD Shed, Gala no 25/26, Ramchandra Bhatt Marg, Next to JJ Hospital Gate no. 2, Opp. Union Bank of India, Noorbaug,
  Mumbai-400009, Maharashtra, India
  Ph: 022-66661880/89   e-mail: mumbai@cbspd.com

Representatives

• Hyderabad	0-9885175004	• Jharkhand	0-9811541605	• Nagpur	0-8692091830
• Patna	0-9334159340	• Pune	0-9664372571	• Uttarakhand	0-9716462459

Printed at Neekunj Print Process, Haryana, India

Forewords

I am glad you have picked up this book because it is designed for today's generation. This book is a primer on charting the perplexed woman. It has the profound insight on woman's health and her health-related problems with their solutions. It is written to enable physiotherapy students, young physiotherapists and women in general to be in tune with pregnancy and postpregnancy physiotherapeutic care.

This text will empower the readers to accelerate knowledge and change their paradigm with crystal clarity. I appreciate the authors Ms. Malti Hiranandani and Ms. Vandana Balaji for their incredibly strategic book and consuming passion for women's health, which compelled them to pen this book straight from experience, knowledge and acquaintance with women patients and students.

Read this book and you will be refined in the field of women's health.

Hannah Rajsekhar (Mrs)
Principal
Apollo College of Physiotherapy
Apollo Hospitals, Hyderabad

It is said that childbirth signifies rebirth of a woman. It brings about a wave of physical and emotional changes in a woman's life. While trying to discover the best ways to care for their children, new (and experienced) mothers often neglect their own health.

This is where a physiotherapist plays a major role in perinatal care, i.e. during and after pregnancy, self-care and baby care.

This book *Physiotherapy in Pregnancy: Antenatal, Postnatal and Baby Care* by two physiotherapists from the Apollo family — Malti Hiranandani and Vandana Balaji — validates the importance of care of self and child, when so much of our society validates neglecting oneself and newborn infant.

It is time that women have access to information that empowers them to nourish and heal themselves and guides them through this vulnerable transition period.

This book makes a perfect gift to any expectant mother. I really appreciate the efforts in writing this book and wish you all success and happiness in life.

Sangita Reddy (Ms)
Director Operations
Apollo Hospitals, Hyderabad

"Women are the real architects of society."

— HARRIET BEECHER STOWE

So very truly said, but ever neglected fact. Women are integral part of our society as a daughter, sister, wife or the mother. A healthy mother nurtures the hopes of a healthy future. This book *Physiotherapy in Pregnancy* focuses on women's health perinatally. I feel proud of the efforts by the two young physiotherapists from our Apollo Hospitals family, Mrs Malti Hiranandani and Mrs Vandana Balaji. They have designed the *Physiotherapy in Pregnancy* to guide all the physiotherapy students, physiotherapists and mothers, today and in future, to improve the women's health and hence lead us to a healthy society.

I wish them all the best in this endeavour and in future.

G. Surender Reddy
CEO & Project Director
Apollo Hospitals, Hyderabad

The stack of information and the bundle of pictures and diagrams define the characteristics of a book and I am glad to pen down words of appreciation for the work of the two authors Ms Malti Hiranandani and Ms Vandana Balaji for their efforts in writing a book with a vision of women's health.

This book *Physiotherapy in Pregnancy* will cater to the needs of a physiotherapy student and the women of today's world. I congratulate them and wish them all success and prosperity in life.

Dr. Hariprasad
Vice-President – Medical Services,
Apollo Hospitals, Hyderabad.

Preface

To woo a man is a woman
To mobilize the world is a woman

I trace myself to the time of evolution and realized that God created man first, that was Adam and when he felt to make Adam complete he made woman that was Eve. It was Eve's womb from where the first seed of life began and there it started the gigantic series of generations which will continue, till the time mankind exists.

Always the *Mankind* is thought of, why not *Womankind*? I know this word does not exist in any English dictionary but it bubbled up in me a couple of years back. I was mesmerized with the responsibilities a physiotherapist can hold in the health of women, when I came across the international standards. During my practice, I was referred women with problems like back pain, knee pain, incontinence, osteoporosis, etc., who were in a wide spectrum of age ranging from 22 to 55 years. Along with their primary problems they had secondary problems which usually remain unfolded and are the causative factor for the vicious cycle of their pain. Secondary problems like mood fluctuations, a weird sense of insecurity and uncontrollable gain in weight come with the package of the woman's body.

Then is a common adage these days that

Men are from Mars and
Women are from Venus.

So I thought, as a physiotherapist I can really be an asset in this world from Mars and can make my Venus world.

With vital support of our colleagues and friends, we began to explore the women's problems, their concerns, the reasoning for their problems and started working up with solutions.

The international market is flooded with a large number of books, videos and CDS for the best health of women but unfortunately we found we are lagging behind.

This competitive element challenged us to work sincerely for the Indian women and our profession too. We are a part of physiotherapy teaching team at Apollo College of Physiotherapy, Apollo Hospitals, Hyderabad. We contemplated that this project will be serving the needs for many.

In this book, we have tried to look from the perspective of a budding physiotherapist, an established physio-therapist, a medical professional, a woman, as well as a lay person interested in the subject.

We have sketched a basic outline of anatomy, physiology, conception, stages of pregnancy, a detailed description of antenatal and postnatal care, and the related common problems faced by a woman. The information given in the text has been practised on patients with satisfactory results.

We hope that readers of this book will be able to have required relevant information and shall be benefited.

Malti Hiranandani
Vandana Balaji

Acknowledgement

Our thoughts are on paper for everybody to read. Our efforts are in black and white to be shared with everybody. We are delighted to bring forward our brainchild which was groomed up by our superiors, colleagues, students and all our near and dear ones.

We take the privilege to thank from the bottom of our hearts our superior, chief and our motivator, Mrs. Hannah Rajsekar, Principal of Apollo College of Physiotherapy.

We extend our gratitude for the valuable contributions by our colleagues, and acknowledge our interns and students, especially for their commitment and kind efforts.

Our special thanks go to expecting and new mothers for sharing their experiences with us and for their active participation in this project.

We extend our thanks to the team of obstetricians and gynecologists of Apollo Hospitals who helped us to treat various women in pregnancy.

We express our sincere thanks to Dr. Pratap C Reddy, Chairman; Mrs. Sangeeta Reddy, Director–Operations; Mr. Surender Reddy, President–Projects; and Dr. Hariprasad, Vice President–Medical Services, Apollo Hospitals, for their constant inspiration and support.

Our sincere and hearty thanks go to Mr Y.N. Arjuna, Publishing Director, CBS, who appreciated our evolving ideas of women's health and groomed them in the form of this book. He weighed our capabilities and enlightened us not just to mark the beginning but showed us a long way to go. Last but not the least, our gratitude is extended to the editing team of CBS Publishers & Distributors for quality inputs.

Malti Hiranandani
Vandana Balaji

Contents

PLATE I

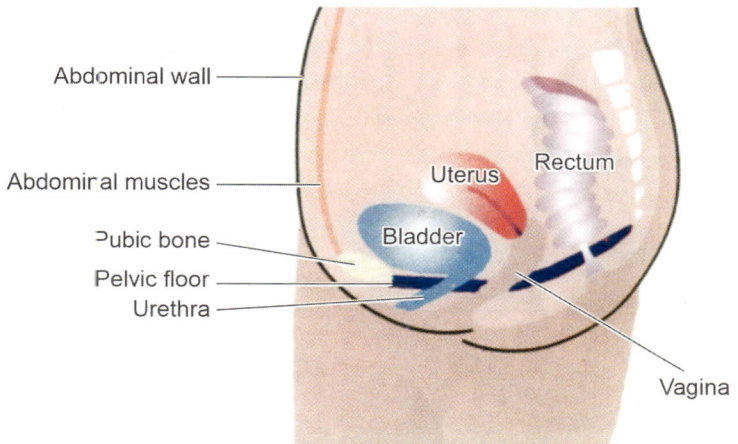

Abdominal wall

Abdomiral muscles

Pubic bone

Pelvic floor

Urethra

Uterus

Rectum

Bladder

Vagina

Fig. 1.1 *Outlook of abdomen*

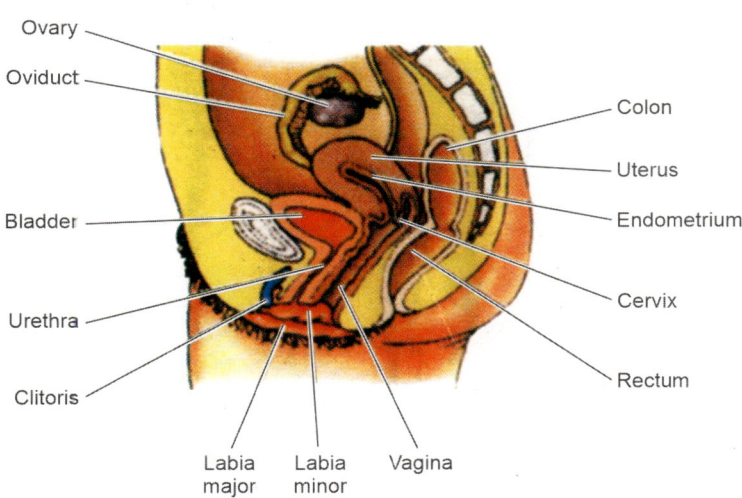

Ovary

Oviduct

Bladder

Urethra

Clitoris

Colon

Uterus

Endometrium

Cervix

Rectum

Labia major

Labia minor

Vagina

Fig. 1.2 *Female reproductive system*

PLATE II

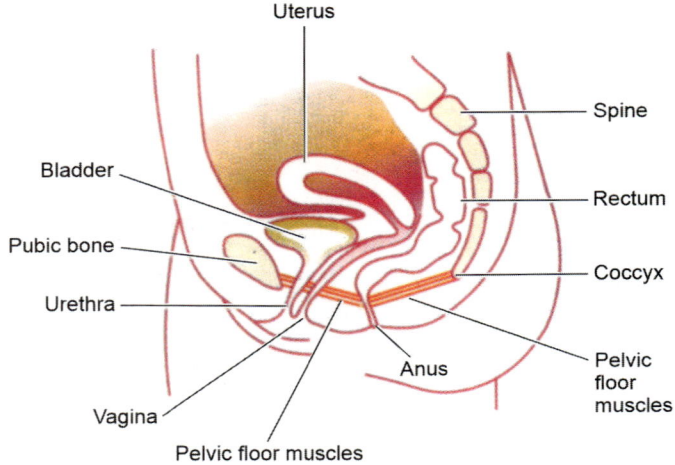

Fig. 1.3 *Pelvic floor region*

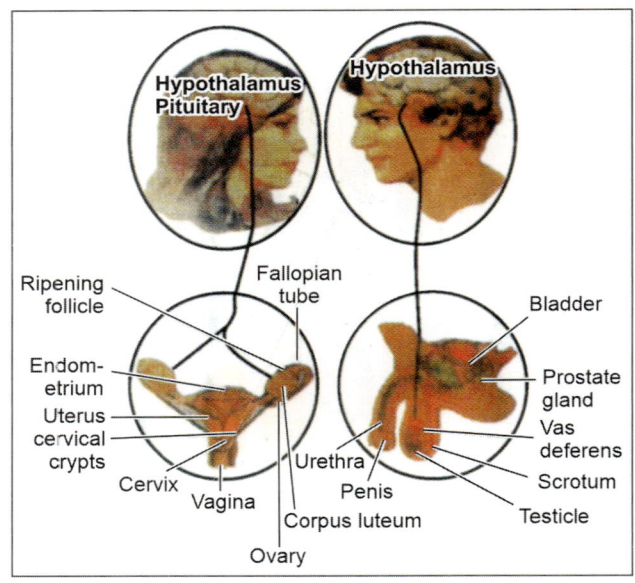

Fig. 1.5 *Regulation of hormones from higher center*

PLATE III

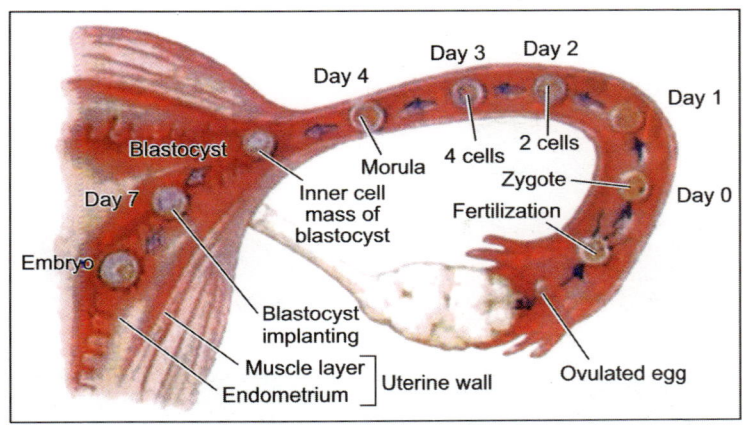

Fig. 2.1 *Stages of maturation of fertilized egg*

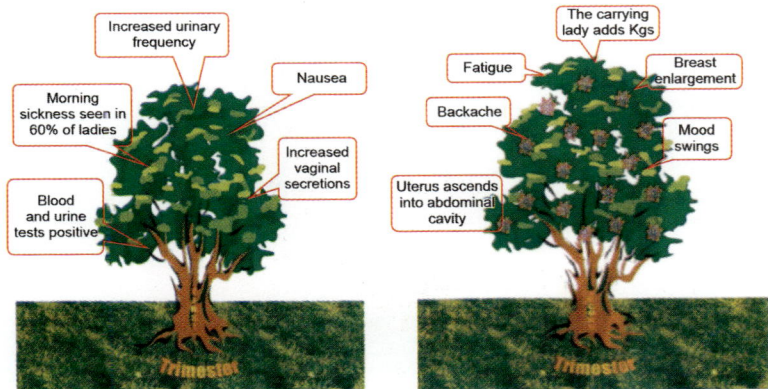

Fig. 3.1 *First trimester of pregnancy with clinical presentations*

Fig. 3.2 *Second trimester of pregnancy with clinical presentations*

PLATE IV

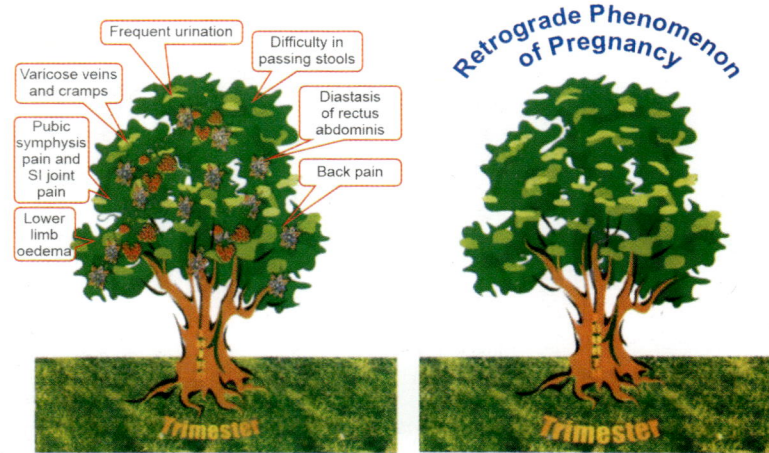

Fig. 3.3 *Third trimester of pregnancy with clinical presentations*

Fig. 3.4 *Fourth trimester of pregnancy with clinical presentations*

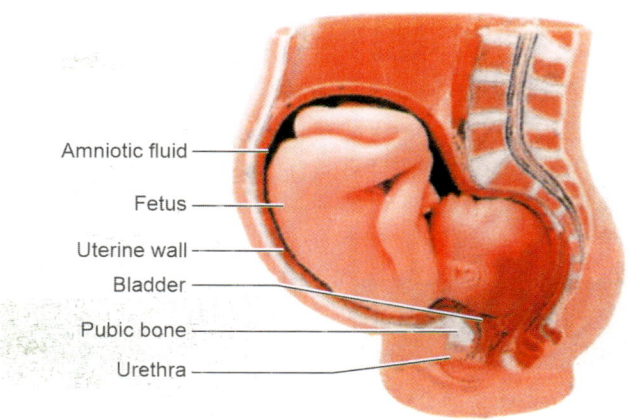

Fig. 3.5 *Ninth month of pregnancy*

PLATE V

Normal anatomy at full term (40 weeks)

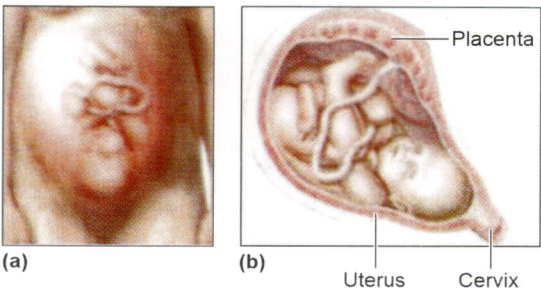

(a) (b)

Placenta

Uterus Cervix

Fig. 9.1 *Demonstrating the position of fetus over the abdomen (a) and in-utero (b)*

Uterus between contractions   Uterus during contractions

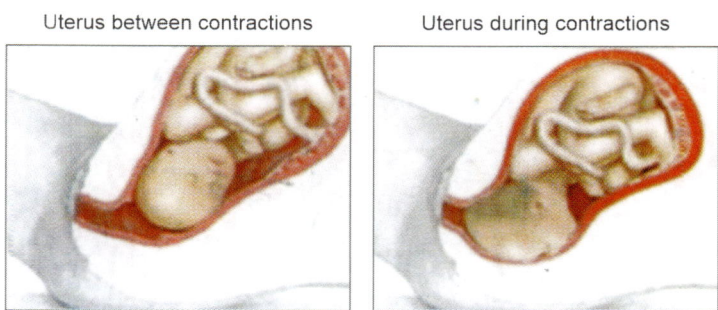

Fig. 9.2 *Uterine contractions*

Undilated, uneffaced   Partly dilated, partly effaced   Fully dilated, fully effaced

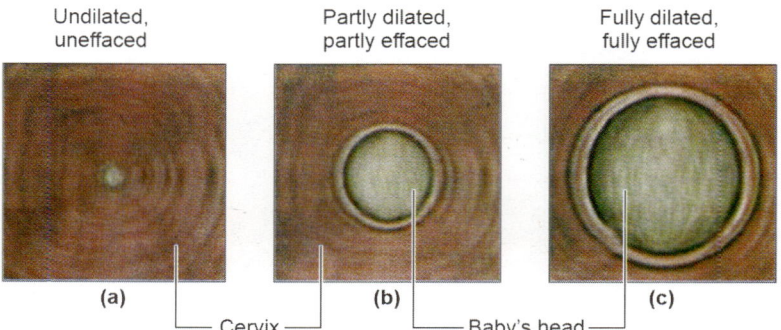

(a) (b) (c)

Cervix   Baby's head

Fig. 9.3 *Dilatation of cervix*

PLATE VI

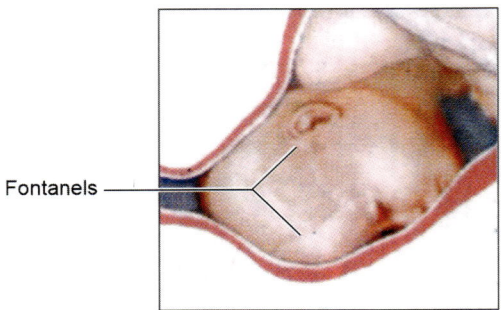

Fig. 9.4 *Foetal fontanels*

Fontanels

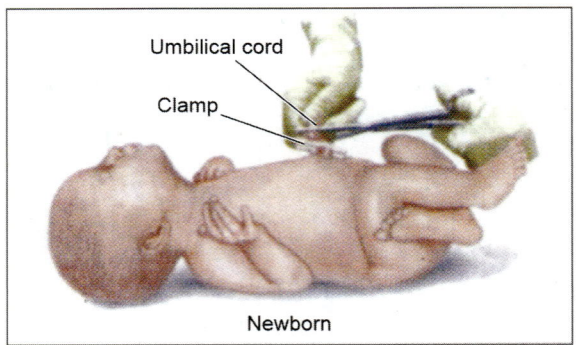

Umbilical cord

Clamp

Newborn

Fig. 9.5 *Newborn baby*

Placenta in uterus
directly after birth

Discharge of placenta

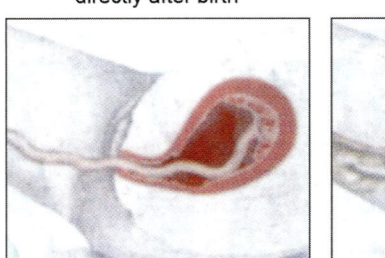
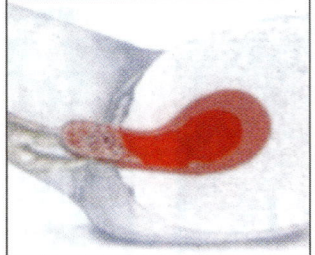

Fig. 9.6 *Placenta discharge*

PLATE VII

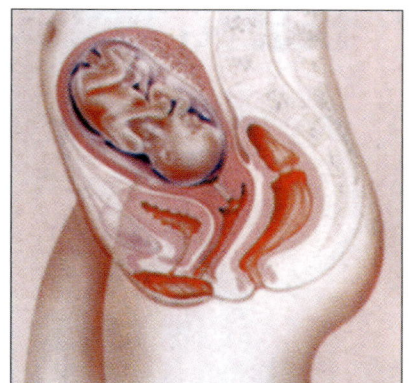

Fig. 9.7 *Foetus position in first stage of labor*

Fetus in breech position

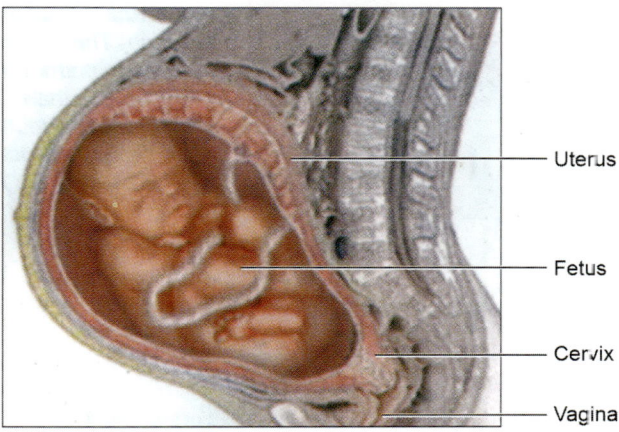

Uterus

Fetus

Cervix

Vagina

Fig. 10.1 *Foetus in breech presentation*

PLATE VIII

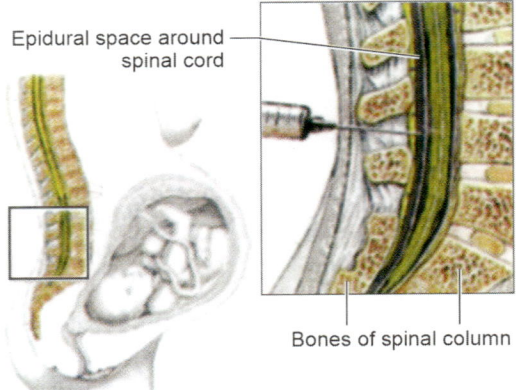

Epidural space around spinal cord

Bones of spinal column

Fig. 10.2 *Spinal/epidural anaesthesia*

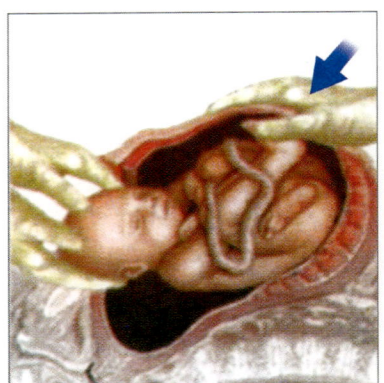

Fig. 10.3 *Caesarean section. The surgeon reaches into the uterus with both hands and lifts the baby's head while the assistant pushes down on the upper uterus to help*

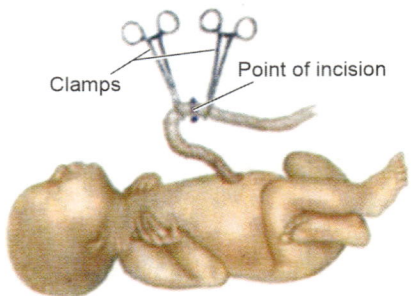

Clamps

Point of incision

Fig. 10.4 *The umbilical cord: The surgeon clamps and cuts the umbilical cord*

Chapter 1
Anatomy and Physiology

ANATOMY OF PELVIS

Pelvis is the base plate of body. It holds the pelvic contents within itself (Fig. 1.1), supports the trunk and helps in transmission of body weight to legs.

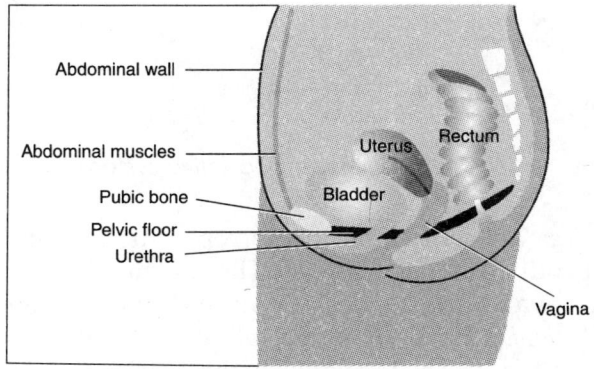

Fig. 1.1 Outlook of abdomen

Pelvis

The pelvis consists of two innominate bones and the sacrum with the coccyx.

These bones articulate at the symphysis pubis at the right angles and at sacroiliac joints to form a bony ring. It is supported by ligaments and muscles.

Female Reproductive Tract

It consists of the following organs: Two ovaries, two fallopian tubes, a uterus and vagina as illustrated in Fig. 1.2.

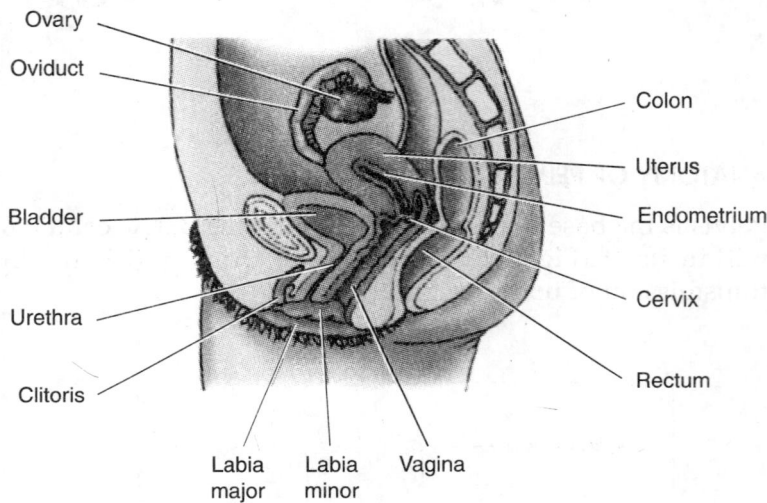

Fig. 1.2 *Female reproductive system*

Ovaries: These are the prime reproductive sex organs which produce female gametes. The function of ovaries is to produce ova and secrete estrogens and progesterone.

The Fallopian tubes: The two fallopian tubes, each 10 cm long, form the connection between the ovaries and the uterus.

The outer end of the tube is funnel-shaped and fimbriated.

The Uterus

It has the following parts:
1. Fundus
2. Body
3. Isthmus
4. Cervix (neck)

It contains myometrium, a thick muscular wall, which is lined with highly vascular endothelium (endometrium).

The neck of uterus forms a canal at the junction of main body of uterus with vagina.

The proximal part of canal is called "internal os". The distal two-thirds protrudes into and forms the vault of vagina. The lowest portion is called the "external os".

Vagina

Normally 7.5 cm long, it is the highly elastic channel. This organ is glandless. It is moistened by transudate and mucus of cervical gland and secretions of uterine endometrium.

The genitalia are divided into external and internal parts.

Internal genitalia are uterus with its appendages and vagina. *External genitalia* are vulva with vaginal openings and openings of vestibular gland.

Supply System

Arterial supply to female reproductive tract is through the left and the right internal iliac arteries. Nerve supply to uterine muscle is by autonomic nervous system via pelvic plexus. Sensory nerve endings are more in cervix and lower uterine segment.

Muscles

Pelvic Floor

⊚ Muscles of pelvis form the floor of perineum and are called pelvic floor muscles. Figure 1.3 shows the position of the pelvic floor muscles.

⊚ Muscles of pelvis are divided into superficial and deep group of muscles.

Superficial Group

External anal sphincter
Ischiocavernosus
Bulbospongiosus
Transversus perinei superficialis

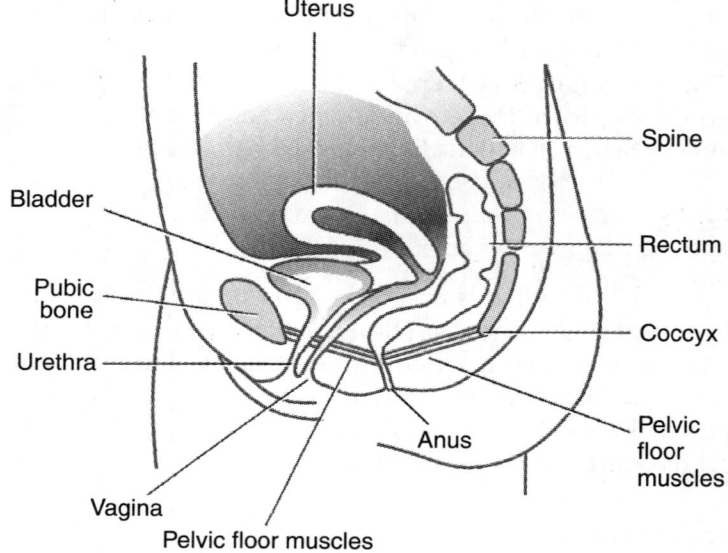

Fig. 1.3 Pelvic floor region

Deep Group

Levator ani
Puborectalis
Pubococcygeus
Iliococcygeus
Ischiococcygeus
Urogenital sphincter

Functions of Pelvic Floor

These are outlined below.

◎ To support the pelvic organs.
◎ To work as an assistance in unloading the spine.
◎ To help in urethral closure during raised intra-abdominal pressure.
◎ To give pelvic–spinal stability.
◎ To control bladder activity.

PHYSIOLOGY

Monthly Cycle

The monthly and rhythmical changes in secretion of female hormones and physical changes corresponding to them are called the *Female monthly sexual cycle or Menstrual cycle*.

The cycle duration is between a time span of 20 days to 45 days but the average number of days is 28. The hormonal fluctuations during the menstrual cycle are shown in a graph in Fig. 1.4.

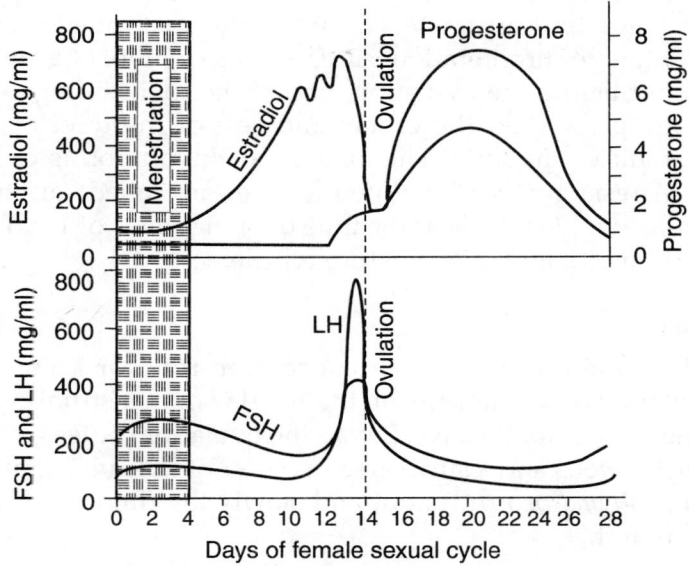

Fig. 1.4 *Hormonal fluctuations during female sexual cycle*

Follicular Phase

This phase starts with *"Primordial follicle"*. This is an ovum with a layer of granulosa cell sheath. After the puberty, under the influence of FSH (follicle stimulating hormone) and LH (luteinizing hormone), follicular growth occurs. Here there is enlargement of ovum with growth of layers of granulosa cells in some follicles. This stage is called *primary follicle*. With this continuous follicular growth in the first few days of the menstrual cycle spindle cells from ovary interstitium proliferate in layers to form a mass called *theca*.

Theca is divided into two layers:

◎ *Theca externa* which forms the capsule of developing follicle.

◎ *Theca interna* is the layer in which the secretion of steroid sex hormones takes place (estrogen and progesterone). In the end phase of proliferation the mass of granulosa cells secretes *follicular fluid* which contains high concentration of estrogen. Accumulation of this fluid causes an Antrum. Vesicular follicles are formed in later stages of proliferation. After a week or more of growth, but before the ovulation, one of the follicles begins to outgrow than the others and rest of the developing follicles involute. This process of Involution is called Atresia and the involuted follicles are called "atretic". The single follicle at the time of ovulation is of 1–1.5 cm in width and it is a mature follicle.

Ovulation

This is the period of high conception rate for a female. Ovulation occurs usually on the 14th day of menstrual cycle, if the cycle is for 28 days. Before the ovulation, outer wall of follicle swells and a small area in center of follicular capsule called *stigma* protrudes out and slowly the fluid oozes out through it.

Corpus Luteum — the Luteal Phase

Under the influence of luteinizing hormone (LH) and follicle-stimulating hormone (FSH) (progesterone), ovulation occurs where the ovum is discharged with the rupture of follicle.

After the expulsion of ovum, remaining granulosa and theca interna cells rapidly change into lutein cell. They get enlarged to two to three folds and get filled with lipids giving them a yellow appearance. This total group of cells is called *corpus luteum* and the process by which it occurs is called *luteinization*.

This corpus luteum grows 1–1.5 cm more in diameter and it is under the secretory zone of progesterone and estrogen. After certain time period say not less than 12 days of ovulation, it is known as *corpus albicans* as it gets involuted, with eventual loss of secretory functions.

Hormonal Action

Gonadotropin hormones FSH and LH are the two active sexual hormones which are the glycoproteins with molecular weights of 30,000. These hormones regulate the sexual cycle, therefore between ages of 11–15 years, when the anterior pituitary gland secretes, these hormones begin *puberty*. The time the first menstrual cycle begins is called *menarche*.

There is regulation of hormonal play both in females and males from the higher centres which is depicted in Fig. 1.5.

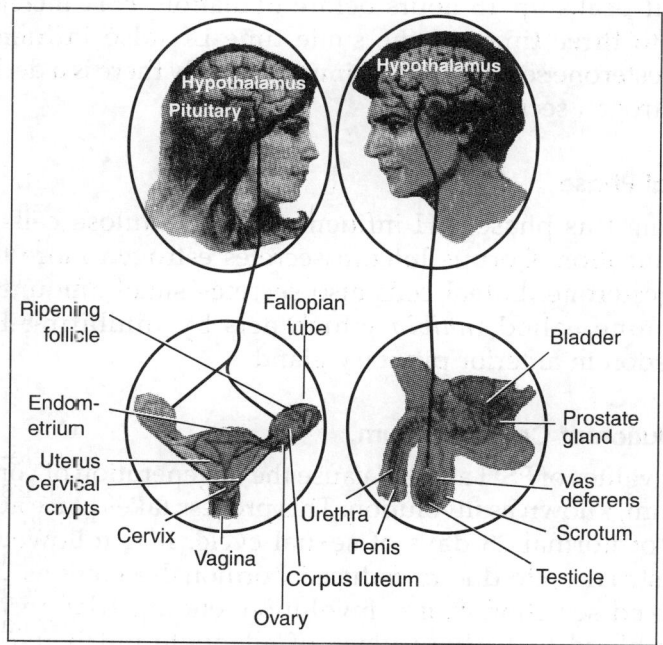

Fig. 1.5 *Regulation of hormones from higher center*

Hormonal Play in Proliferative/Estrogen Phase/Follicular Phase

Under the influence of large quantities of FSH and LH, the entire ovaries with some follicles within them begin to grow. Slowly FSH exceeds LH secretion, which causes increase in growth of 6–12 primary follicles each month. Estrogen in huge amounts from fastest growing follicle act on hypothalamus to depress the further secretion of FSH by anterior pituitary gland and thereby inhibits the further growth of less developed follicles. Therefore, only a single follicle reaches for ovulation.

Ovulation—High Surge of LH/Secretory Phase/ Progestational Phase

LH secretion enhances usually two days before ovulation and it peaks up 16 hours before ovulation. FSH increases two to three times at the same time LH also influences progesterone secretion, and simultaneously there is a decline in estrogen secretion.

Luteal Phase

During this phase, LH influences the granulosa cells for luteinization. Corpus luteum secretes estrogen more than progesterone. Luteal cells also secretes small amounts of hormone called *inhibin* which acts by inhibiting FSH secretion in anterior pituitary gland.

Involution of Corpus Luteum

Low values of FSH and LH cause the degeneration of corpus luteum, known as involution. This process takes place at 26th day of normal 28 days of sexual cycle. It is followed by menstrual cycle due to reduced hormonal secretions. This reduced secretion causes involution, endometrial necrosis with blood loss (due to lack of adequate nutrients) and vasospasm.

A new ovarian cycle follows, where slowly there is a rise in FSH and LH- initiating, growth of new follicles.

Capacitation

This is a process, where sperm and ovum are provided with external nutrients in the fallopian tube to get fertilized and result in the formation of zygote.

Chapter 2

Pregnancy and Hormonal Play

PREGNANCY

Maturation and Fertilization of the Ovum

In the ovary the ovum is in the primary oocyte stage. Before getting released from the ovarian follicle, nucleus divides by meiosis and a first polar body is expelled, where the primary oocyte becomes the secondary oocyte, where each of the 23 pairs of chromosomes loses one of its partners which becomes incorporated in a polar body that is expelled, which leaves 23 unpaired chromosomes in the secondary oocyte.

At this juncture, ovum which is in the secondary oocyte stage is ovulated into the abdominal cavity and then immediately it enters the fallopian tube.

Entry of Ovum into the Oviduct

Corona radiata is the ovum along with hundreds of granulosa cells. When ovulation occurs corona radiata is expelled into peritoneal cavity and enters one of the fallopian tubes to reach the uterus.

The Semen and Fertilization of Ovum

Almost half a billion sperms are deposited in the vagina.

After ejaculation, few a sperms are transported within 5 to 10 minutes upward from the vagina and through the uterus and fallopian tubes, to reaches the ampullae of the fallopian tubes.

Transportation of the sperm is aided by contraction of the uterus and fallopian tubes that are stimulated by prostaglandins in the male seminal fluid and also by oxytocin of the female during orgasm. Fertilization takes place in the ampulla of one of the fallopian tubes.

Sperm has to penetrate corona radiata. Once sperm has entered the ovum, oocyte divides to form a mature ovum and a second polar body is expelled. The mature ovum undergoes the stages of zygote, morula, blastocyte and finally the embryo. Figure 2.1 shows the stages of maturation of fertilised egg.

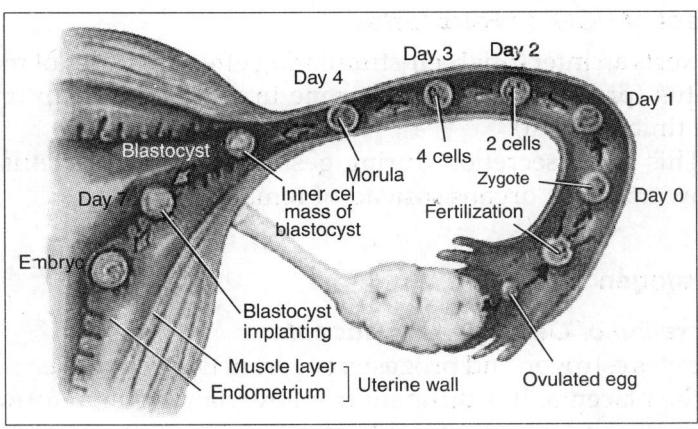

Fig. 2.1 *Stages of maturation of fertilized egg*

ROLE OF HORMONES

Human Chorionic Gonadotropin

Human chorionic gonadotropin (HCG) is a glycoprotein. It causes persistence of corpus luteum and also prevents menstruation. It is secreted by syncytial trophoblast cells into the fluids of mother and in newly developing embryonic tissues.

The rate of secretion of HCG rises rapidly to reach maximum at about 10 to 12 weeks and decreases to a lower value by 16 to 20 weeks and continues at this rate for the rest of the pregnancy.

Functions of HCG

The functions of HCG are:
1. To prevent involution of corpus luteum at the end of the monthly female sexual cycle.
2. Causes corpus luteum to secrete even larger quantities of its sex hormones, i.e. progesterone, estrogen for the next few months.

Effect of HCG on Fetal Testes

It exerts an interstitial cell-stimulating effect on testes of male foetus (production of testosterone in male fetuses up until the time of birth)

This small secretion during gestation causes the fetus to grow male sex organs instead of female organs.

Oestrogen

Secretion of Oestrogen by Placenta

Secretes estrogen and progesterone from the trophoblast cells of the placenta. It is different from ovarian estrogen formed from the androgenic steroid compounds (adrenal glands).

Functions of Estrogen in Pregnancy

1. Enlargement of mother's uterus.
2. Enlargement of mother's breasts and growth of breast ductal structure.
3. Enlargement of mother's female external genitalia.
4. Relax the pelvic ligaments of mother, so that sacroiliac (SI) joint becomes relatively limber and symphysis pubis becomes elastic, which makes easier passage of the fetus through birth canal.
5. Also affects the rate of cell production in early embryo.

Secretion of Progesterone by the Placenta

◎ Moderate quantities are produced by corpus luteum in the beginning of the pregnancy.
◎ Later on, tremendous quantities by placenta are produced.
◎ Ten- fold increase during the course of pregnancy.

Progesterone

Effects of Progesterone

1. Causes decidual cells to develop in the uterine endometrium and play an important role in nutrition of early embryo.
2. Decreases contractility of pregnant uterus preventing contractions from causing spontaneous abortion.
3. It provides nutritive material for developing morula and blastocytes even before its implantation.
4. Helps the estrogen to prepare the mother's breasts for lactation.

Human Chorionic Somatomammotropin

Human chorionic somatomammotropin is a protein. Recently discovered placental hormone is a general metabolic hormone that has specific nutritional implications for both mother and fetus.

OTHER HORMONAL FACTORS IN PREGNANCY

Pituitary Secretions

◎ The anterior pituitary gland of mother enlarges at least 50% during pregnancy and increases its production of corticotropin, thyrotropin and prolactin. FSH, LH are suppressed totally due to inhibiting effects of oestrogen and progesterone from the placenta.
◎ Corticosteroid secretion:
◎ Secretions from the thyroid gland: During pregnancy, usually enlarges up to 50% and there is an increased production of thyroxine.

Partly the secretion of thyroxine is influenced by HCG and HCT (human chorionic thyrotropin-secreted by placenta).

Corticosteroid Secretions

◎ There is a moderate increase in glucocorticoids through out pregnancy. They are responsible to mobilise amino acids from the mother's tissues, which can be used for the synthesis of tissues in foetus.

◎ Throughout the course of pregnancy, about twin-fold increase in aldosterone is present which reaches its peak at the end of gestation.

Aldosterone and oestrogen causes the reabsorption of excess sodium from renal tubules of the mother, and retains fluid occasionally leading to Pregnancy Hypertension.

Thyroid Gland Secretions

There is a 50% enlargement of the thyroid gland during pregnancy and corresponding increase in the production of thyroxine.

Parathyroid Gland Secretions

When the mother is on a calcium-deficient diet, there is usually enlargement of this gland. It is even more intensified during lactation as a growing baby's calcium requirements are higher.

Secretions of Relaxin by the Ovaries and the Placenta

Relaxin is a polypeptide and is secreted by corpus luteum of the ovary and by placental tissues. It is increased by the stimulating effect of human chorionic gonadotropin, at the same time when estrogen and progesterone are secreted in corpus luteum and in the placenta.

Relaxin helps in the softening the cervix of the pregnant woman at the time of delivery.

PARTURITION (BIRTH OF A BABY)

The uterus becomes more excitable until finally it develops strong rhythmic contractions and with that force the baby is expelled out. The causes for increased intense contractions for parturition are as follows.

Hormonal Changes that Cause Increased Excitability of the Uterine Musculature.

- Ratio of oestrogen to progesterone
- The role of progesterone is to inhibit uterine contractility during pregnancy, in turn helping to prevent expulsion of foetus.
- The role of oestrogen is to increase degree of uterine contractility.

Both the hormones are secreted in progressively greater quantities throughout and from the 7th month onwards oestrogen increases while progesterone remains constant/ decreases slightly.

Effects of Oxytocin on Uterus

The role of oxytocin is specific for uterine contractions.
- The oxytocin receptors in the uterine musculature increases.
- The secretion increases at the time of labour.

Effect of Foetal Hormones on Uterus

- The pituitary gland of foetus secretes increasing quantities of oxytocin which plays a role in exciting the uterus.
- The adrenal glands secrete large quantities of cortisone which help in uterine contractions.
- The foetal membrane releases prostaglandins in high concentration at the time of labour which intensifies the uterine contractility.

Mechanical Factors which Increase the Contractility of the Uterus

Stretch of the Uterine Musculature

Stretching of the smooth muscle organs increase the contractility. In the process of parturition there is intermittent stretch in the uterus due to the movement of the foetus.

The importance of mechanical stretch in eliciting uterine contraction is emphasized in the birth of twins who are born 19 days prior than a single child.

Stretch/irritation of the Cervix

Stretching or irritation of the nerves in the cervix initiates reflexes to the body of the uterus which in turn increases uterine contractility and also myogenic transmission of signals from cervix to body of uterus.

PREGNANCY AND ITS EFFECT ON SYSTEMS

Gastrointestinal System

Peristalsis movements may reduce and the lady may show symptoms of nausea and vomiting. Therefore, the lady is advised to stop eating heavy meals at one time, rather prefer short, frequent light meals.

Cardiovascular Systems

1. The characteristic change is seen in plasma levels, where they shoot up in comparison with red blood cells leading to 'physiological anemia'. This is also called as *'pregnancy anemia'*, as it is due to raised plasma volumes which are in response to hormonal changes, in order to meet high oxygen demands.
2. There is increase in heart size, heart rate and cardiac output. Heart rate increases 10–20 beats/min and so, there is an increase in cardiac output of 30–60%.
3. The increased uterine size and venous distensibility causes increased venous pressure in lower limbs.

4. Blood pressure changes are variable during the three trimesters. It is at low levels in first trimester, lowest in the second trimester, and then there is gradual rise in the third trimester, till six weeks postdelivery.

The blood-pressure swings between pushings and contractions during labour. It moves like a sea wave, where it rises with pushings and falls with contractions. In labour, if the lady, holds her breath for prolonged time while bearing down, which is strictly not advisable, then it raises intra-thoracic and intra-abdominal pressure, which in turn leads to venous compression and blocks return of blood to heart. Therefore, cardiac output shoots down as well as blood pressure levels.

Respiratory System

1. There is rise in anteroposterior and transverse diameter of chest by 2 cm.
2. As the ribs flare up and out due to hormone stimulation, diaphragm gets elevated by 4 cm.
3. Respiratory rate does not change much but, definitely there is an increase in depth of respiration.
4. Tidal volume increases, with not so much marked changes in total lung capacity.
5. To meet the high oxygen demands during pregnancy, the lady is usually in a state of hyperventilation.

During labour, the state of hyperventilation is more prominent, specially in the 1st stage, where respiratory rate and depth increases in response to increased oxygen requirement. There is a decline in arterial PCO_2 levels usually during labour. If the woman does overbreathing, it can make her blood alkalotic. This alkalosis leads to reduced oxygen being more tightly attached to heamoglobin and thereby, resulting in its reduced availability. In this case, oxygen depletion occurs in fetal circulation leading to fetal distress.

Thermoregulatory System

1. Hike in the BMR and heat production during pregnancy.

2. A load of 300 kilocalories/day becomes the requisite to meet the high body demands.
3. During labour the lady feels very hot and profuse sweating, due to strong muscle activity with production of heat.

Musculoskeletal System

1. The constant growing weight of foetus and hormonal changes affects the ligaments and muscles leading to their increased laxity and joint hypermobility.
2. By the last trimester of pregnancy, abdominal muscles are stretched to the maximum point of its elastic limit.
3. The constant growing weight of foetus and hormonal changes affects the ligaments and muscles leading to their increased laxity and joint hypermobility.
4. By the last trimester of pregnancy, abdominal muscles are stretched to maximum point of its elastic limit.

FERTILE PHASE OF A FEMALE

Identification by Self

1. Cervical mucus is an important indicator of fertility.
   The mucus is produced by cervical crypts and is of two types.
   i. Estrogen-based thin type
   ii. Progesterone-based thick type

Oestrogen-Based Thin Type

The estrogen based mucus is:
   a. Clear, thin, slippery and stretchy like the raw white of the egg.
   b. Enables sperm movements freely into the uterus.
   c. Stretches about two inches without breaking.
   d. Protects the sperms by enveloping them.
   e. Filters out damaged sperms.

Progesterone-Based Thick Type

Progesterone alters the mucus which becomes thick, turbid and sticky. It is difficult for the sperms to penetrate and be-transported up

2. In cervical mucus, sperm can survive for 3 days or more where it is fertile.

3. The fertile period is all the wet days and 3 days are added to it.

4. Checking the temperature every day morning the body temperature is checked before brushing.

   Secretion of progesterone during the later half of the cycle, raises the body temperature about 0.5 degree Fahrenheit, the temperature raise coming abruptly at the time of the ovulation.

5. Other ways of checking the fertile period are the recent advancement of the hormonal studies.

   Follicular study helps in identifying the maturation of the ovum and rupture.

Chapter 3

Pregnancy—Week By Week

The unborn baby spends around 38 weeks in the womb, but the average length of pregnancy (gestation) is counted as 40 weeks. This is because pregnancy is counted from the first day of the woman's last period, not the date of conception, which generally occurs two weeks later. Pregnancy is divided into the following three trimesters (Figs 3.1 to 3.4).

First trimester - conception to 12 weeks

Second trimester - 12 to 24 weeks

Third trimester - 24 to 40 weeks

Figures 3.1, 3.2, 3.3 and 3.4 show the stages of pregnancy with their clinical presentations.

Conception

The moment of conception is when the woman's ovum (egg) is fertilized by the man's sperm. The gender and inherited characteristics are decided in that instant.

PREGNANCY—WEEKLY DEVELOPMENT

Week 1

Thirty hours after conception, the cell splits into two. By day 3, the cell (*zygote*) has divided into 16 cells. After two more days, the zygote has migrated from the fallopian tube to the uterus. At day 7, the zygote burrows itself into the plump uterine lining (endometrium). The zygote is now known as a *blastocyst*.

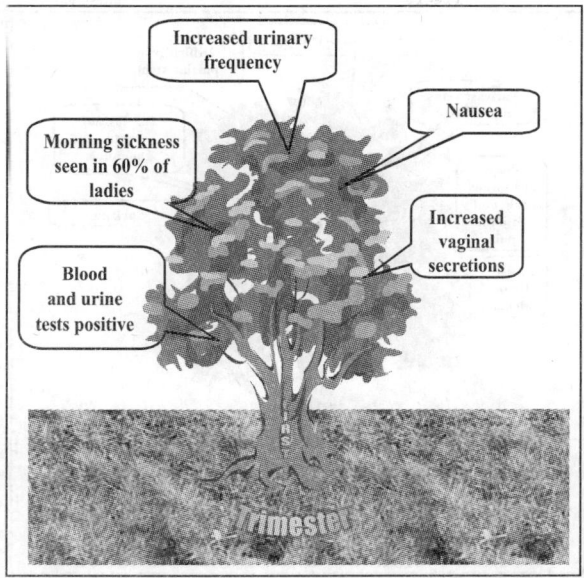

Fig. 3.1 *First trimester of pregnancy with clinical presentations*

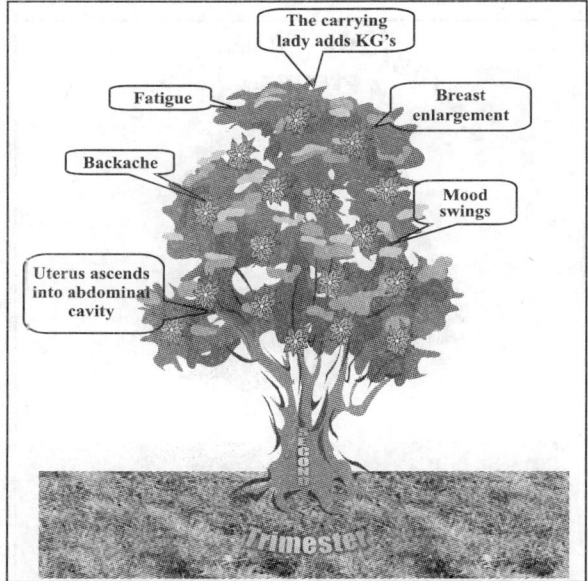

Fig. 3.2 *Second trimester of pregnancy with clinical presentations*

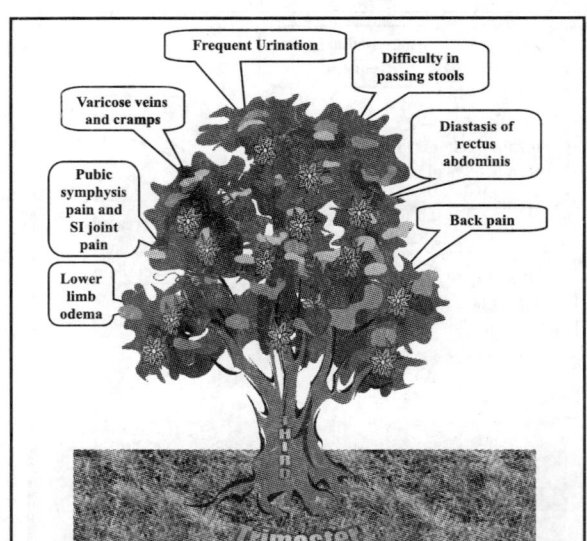

Fig. 3.3 *Third trimester of pregnancy with clinical presentations*

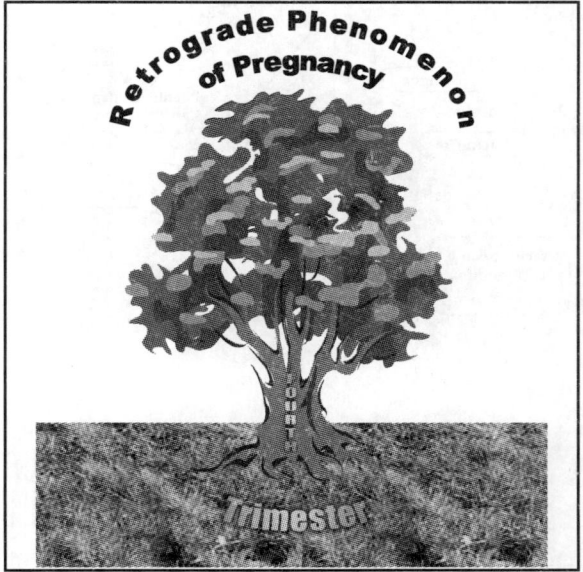

Fig. 3.4 *Fourth trimester of pregnancy with clinical presentations*

Week 2

The developing baby is tinier than a grain of rice. The rapidly dividing cells are in the process of forming the various body systems, including the digestive system.

Week 3

The evolving neural tube will eventually become the central nervous system (brain and spinal cord).

Week 4

The baby is now known as an embryo. It is around 3 mm in length. By this stage, it is secreting special hormones that prevent the mother from having a menstrual period.

Week 5

The heart starts beating. The embryo has developed its placenta and amniotic sac. The placenta is burrowing into the uterine wall to access oxygen and nutrients from the mother's bloodstream.

Week 6

The embryo is now around 1.3 cm in length. The rapidly growing spinal cord looks like a tail. The head is disproportionately large.

Week 7

The eyes, mouth and tongue are forming. The tiny muscles allow the embryo to start moving about. Blood cells are being made by the embryo's liver.

Week 8

The embryo is now known as a foetus and is about 2.5 cm in length. All of the body organs are formed. The hands and feet, which previously looked like nubs or paddles, are now evolving into fingers and toes. The brain is active, and has brain waves.

Week 9

Teeth are budding inside the gums. The tiny heart is developing further.

Week 10

The fingers and toes are recognizable, but still stuck together with webs of skin.

Week 11

The foetus can swim about quite vigorously. It is now more than 7 cm in length.

Week 12

The eyelids are fused over the fully developed eyes. The baby can now mutely cry, since it has vocal cords. It may even start sucking its thumb. The fingers and toes are growing nails.

Week 13

The muscles develop further, and the baby's movements as it swims and kicks are more coordinated.

Week 16

The foetus is around 14 cm in length. Eyelashes and eyebrows have appeared, and the tongue has tastebuds. An ultrasound is commonly performed around this time (usually week 18) to check for abnormalities, position of placenta and multiple pregnancies. Interestingly, hiccoughs in the foetus can often be observed.

Week 20

The foetus is around 21 cm in length. The ears are fully functioning and can hear muffled sounds from the outside world. The fingertips have prints. The genitals can now be distinguished with an ultrasound scan.

Week 24

The foetus is around 33 cm in length. The fused eyelids now separate into upper and lower lids, enabling the baby to open and shut its eyes. The skin is covered in fine hair (lanugo) and protected by a layer of waxy secretion (vernix). The baby 'breathes' amniotic fluid in and out of its lungs.

Week 28

The foetus is around 37 cm in length. The growing body has caught up with the large head, and the baby now seems more in proportion.

Week 32

The baby spends most of its time asleep. Its movements are strong and coordinated. It has probably assumed the 'head down' position by now, in preparation for birth.

Week 36

The baby is around 46 cm in length. It has probably nestled its head into its mother's pelvis, ready for birth. If it is born now, its chances for survival are excellent. Development of the lungs is rapid over the next few weeks.

Week 38

The baby is around 51 cm in length and ready to be born. It is thought that the baby secretes hormones that trigger the onset of labour. Figure 3.5 shows the position of the baby in the ninth month of pregnancy.

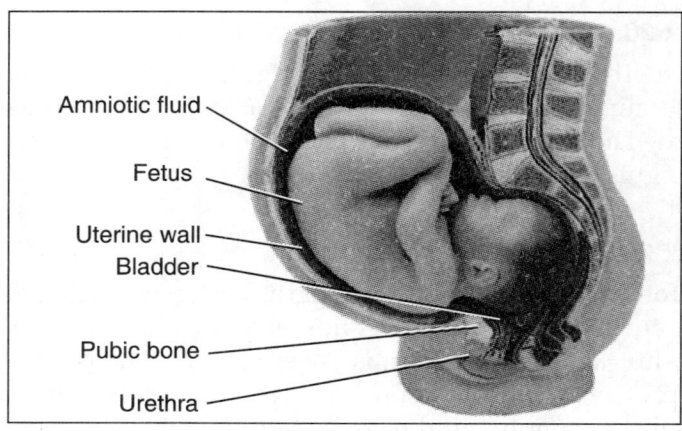

Amniotic fluid

Fetus

Uterine wall

Bladder

Pubic bone

Urethra

Fig. 3.5 Ninth month of pregnancy

Chapter 4

Assessment

The Physiotherapist's
GYNAECOLOGICAL ASSESSMENT

Name:
Age:
Occupation
Marital status: Years of marriage
Last menstruation date
Pregnancy status: Number of pregnancies
Expected delivery Date

History:
    Any previous medical/ surgical/family history
    Any previous obstetrical/gynaecological history
    Number of pregnancies and child status
    Types of delivery: episiotomy/C-section/ forceps/ normal.
    Any abortions: Miscarriages / MTP

Present status:
    Complains of the patient: Morning sickness/dizziness
        Swelling of legs
        Pain in back/neck/wrist
        Night cramps

The Physiotherapist's Gynaecological Assessment

General Examination
  Height
  Weight
  Vitals
    Temperature
    Blood pressure
    Heart rate
    Respiratory rate
    Pallor/oedema
    Posture

Pain Evaluation

Site

Duration

Type (McGill Melnack Pain Questionnaire)

Level (VAS-Visual Analogue Scale)

Visual analogue Scale

Describe the discomfort or pain on a scale of 0 to 10

N one	Mild		Moderate				Severe	
1	2	3	4	5	6	7	8	9	10

Range of movement (ROM)—upper limb and lower limb

Muscle strength assessment (Oxford Scale)
  Bilateral—upper limb
  Bilateral—lower limb
  Pelvic floor

Any tightness / contracture / deformity

Any relevant investigations
  Blood profile
  Urinary status
  Ultrasound

Psychosocial status

Any other complains (like gestational diabetes, incontinence)

Physiotherapy goals
  Short-term goals
  Long-term goals

Physiotherapy management

Patients are asked to underline not more than one word from any or all of the 20 groups which best describe their pain. The simplest scoring methods involve:

◎ Total number of words underlined

◎ Intensity, measured by allotting score 1 to the first word in any group, 1 to the second, and so on.

◎ The first 10 groups are somatic (describing what the pain feels like)

◎ 11 to 15 are affective

◎ 16 is evaluative

◎ 17 to 20 are miscellaneous

The McGill Melnack Pain Questionnaire (Ref: Sullivan et al)

Group 1	Group 2	Group 3	Group 4	Group 5
Flickering	Jumping	Pricking	Sharp	Pinching
Quivering	Flashing	Boring	Gritting	Pressing
Pulsing	Shooting	Drilling	Lacerating	Gnawing
Throbbing		Stabbing		Cramping
Beating		Lancinating		Crushing
Pounding				

Group 6	Group 7	Group 8	Group 9	Group 10
Tugging	Hot	Tingling	Dull	Tender
Pulling	Burning	Itching	Sore	Taut
Wrenching	Scalding	Smarting	Hurting	Rasping
	Searing	Stinging	Aching	Splitting
			Heavy	

Group 11	Group 12	Group 13	Group 14	Group 15
Tiring	Sickening	Fearful	Punishing	Wretched
Exhausting	Suffocating	Frightful	Gruelling	Blinding
		Terrifying	Cruel	
			Vicious	
			Killing	

Group 16	Group 17	Group 18	Group 19	Group 20
Annoying	Spreading	Tight	Cool	Nagging
Trouble-	Radiating	Numb	Cold	Nau-
some				seating
Miserable	Penetra-	Drawing	Freezing	Agonizing
	ting			
Intense	Piercing	Squeezing		Dreadful
Unbearable		Tearing		Torturing

Chapter 5

Antenatal Care

ANTENATAL CARE

Guidelines for Exercises in Pregnancy

1. Consult the doctor before commencing exercises.
2. Gradually increases the dosage of exercises especially if the lady is not a regular exercise doing person.
3. Exercises are done regularly three times a week.
4. Maximum heart rate should not exceed 140–150 beats/minute during the exercises.
5. Moderate period of exercise should not exceed duration of 20 minutes.
6. Ensure adequate warm-up and cool-down periods.
7. Maintain adequate fluid intake to avoid dehydration
8. Avoid exercises in supine after end of 4 month.
9. Avoid contact sports after 16 weeks gestation.
10. Avoid ballistic bounces with stretches.
11. Avoid stretching in extreme ranges of movement.
12. Avoid Valsalva's maneuver during exercise.

Benefits of Exercise in Pregnancy

1. Maintains cardiovascular fitness
2. Improves circulation
3. Maintains muscle length and flexibility
4. Strengthens specific muscles required during pregnancy period and labour
5. Improves breath awareness and control
6. Increases endurance
7. Improves coordination, balance and rhythm

8. Reinforces the principles of relaxation
9. Decreases physical problems like nausea, backache.
10. Reduces stress and anxiety
11. Provides social interaction.

Contraindications to Exercises

1. Women with diseases of cardiovascular, respiratory or renal systems.
2. Diabetic women or women with thyroid disease. Women with history of miscarriage, premature labour, cervical incompetence in multiple pregnancies.
3. Vaginal bleeding or fluid loss, hypertensive women.
4. Abnormal placental function or position, decreased foetal movements.
5. Breech presentation in third trimester should not go for exercises.
6. Women with anemia or other blood disorders.

Risk of Intensive Exercises

1. Risk of musculoskeletal trauma due to connective tissue laxity.
2. Risk of increased demand on cardiovascular system.
3. Hypoglycaemia could be a very common complaint.
4. Foetal distress.
5. Intrauterine growth retardation can be a major risk.
6. Foetal malformation due to increased maternal core
7. Preterm labour with or without delivery is commonly seen in women who do not do exercises.

Potential Risk to Foetus from Maternal Exercises

1. Hyperthermia.
2. Hypoxia
3. Abnormal heart rate
4. Decreased uteroplacental flow.
5. Increased uterine contractions.
6. Reduced maternal glucose levels

7. Disruption of maternal endocrine haemostasis.
8. Poor growth of foetus.

Aims of Antenatal Care

1. To give necessary information about pregnancy, labour stages, delivery and postdelivery sequences.
2. To encourage the lady to maintain her optimum physical and mental health.
3. To plan out child-care program.
4. To prevent medical or obstetrics complications and if it happens the management for same.

Physiotherapy Sessions

To organize physiotherapy sessions, we require the following.
1. Small group (8–10 pregnant ladies)
2. Well ventilated rooms
3. Soft slow music
4. Carpeted supportive floor
5. Large mirrors for visual feedback
6. Equipped with emergency equipment

ANTENATAL CLASSES

The classes which are conducted during the nine months of gestation are called antenatal classes. Usually three to four sessions are taken for a group of 3–5 couples.

These sessions are preferred in the second trimester where three sessions are conducted and the last session is done in the beginning of third trimester.

Division of Sessions

First Session

Introduction of couples to each other and a video/slide show which guides them about the anatomy, physiology and significance of exercises in the pregnancy.

Second Session

To start the antenatal care the lady is taught first relaxation and breathing exercises in first level of antenatal class. Demonstration and practice of breathing, relaxation, general body, stretching and strengthening exercises in a group.

Third Session

Kegel exercises, abdominal and spinal extension exercises, posture care. Do's and dont's to be followed.

Fourth Session

Stages of labour, exercises in the stages, coping strategies of labour, baby care tips. They are also known as **Lamaze classes.**

BREATHING EXERCISES

These are performed to improve pulmonary status, promote relaxation, enhance overall endurance and functional potential.

Breathing Exercises Preparation

A well ventilated room. A comfortable and relaxed position where person usually adopts a Crook lying position (head and trunk elevated to 45 degrees, hips and knees flexed, with a pillow supporting the legs). This position is mostly the line of choice. Sitting, standing or lying are also other options.

DIAPHRAGMATIC BREATHING

Diaphragm is the main muscle of inspiration. Accessory muscles are trapezius, scaleni, levator scapulae and sternocleidomastoid.

To teach the pregnant lady diaphragmatic breathing, she is advised first to be in crook lying position (explained earlier). The neck, scapulae, and head region should be relaxed. The physiotherapist places her hand on the belly (rectus abdominis), below the anterior costal margin, and asks the lady to inhale slowly and deeply through nose. The therapist's hands are superimposed with the lady's hand, so when 'the would be' mother inhales, her belly will rise up and then she slowly exhales through her mouth. Figure 5.1 shows the positioning for performing the diaphragmatic breathing exercises.

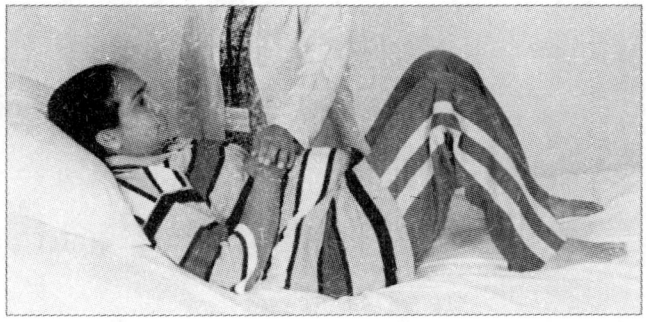

Fig. 5.1 *Diaphragmatic breathing*

The therapist can explain the same exercise with the example of a balloon.

Where the balloon gets bloated when air is driven into it and flattens when air is expelled out.

Once the mother-to-be masters this technique she is advised to do the same exercise in standing, sitting and during her daily activities.

SEGMENTAL BREATHING

The upper middle and lower segments are individually expanded through the means of breathing exercises. The basic mechanism remains the same as explained above only the position of the hand varies.

Upper/Apical

Therapist's hands are placed over the clavicle superimposed with the lady's hand and instructions are to take deep breaths in through nose and out through mouth, using the accessory muscles (Fig. 5.2).

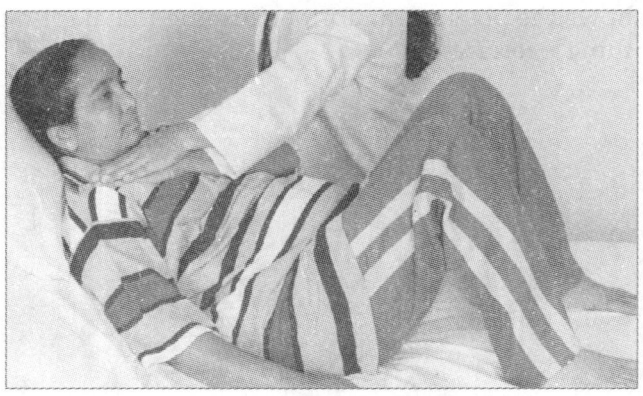

Fig. 5.2 *Apical breathing*

Middle Segment

Therapists hands are placed, either unilaterally/ bilaterally on the sides of the chest (rib cage) just below the axilla (as shown in Fig. 5.3), superimposed with lady' hand and same instructions are given, i.e. to breathe in through nose and breathe out through mouth.

RELAXATION

A healthy physical and mental status makes an individual relaxed. Therefore, for relaxation the initial steps to follow are as follows.

1. Quiet, cozy place.
2. Well ventilated room/ open space.
3. Area to be free of noise or a gentle soothing music.
4. Loose, comfortable garments.

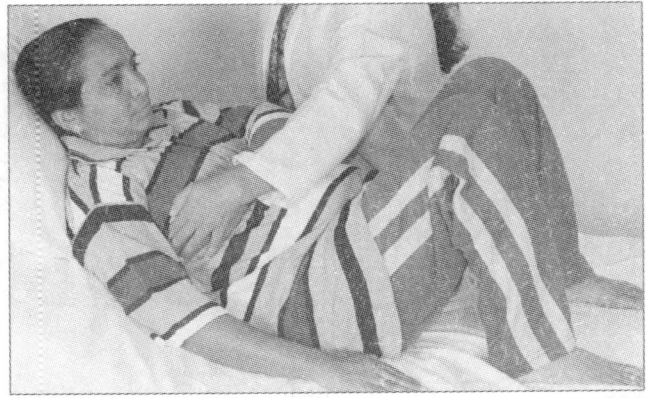

Fig. 5.3 *Lateral costal breathing*

Deep breathing, different meditation techniques, warm touch of therapist/partner help in giving relaxation to the pregnant lady.

Savasana position: Supine position, lying with legs straight, arms abducted and extended is commonly the adopted posture by tensed individuals as seen in Fig. 5.4.

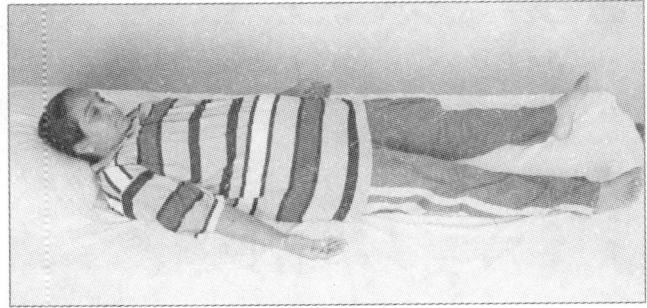

Fig. 5.4 *Savasana*

Other different positions to practice are as follows.
a. Lying with pillows under head and pillows under knees in flexion as seen in Fig. 5.5.

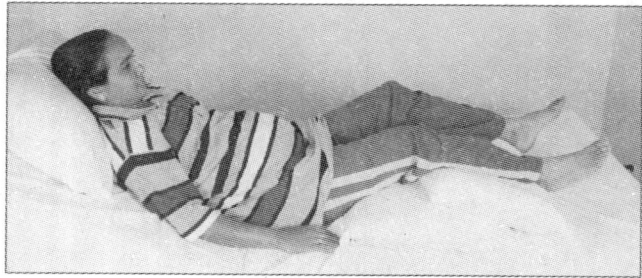

Fig. 5.5 Relaxed – half lying position

b. Side lying with pillow under head and under flexed knees as depicted in Figs 5.6 and 5.7.

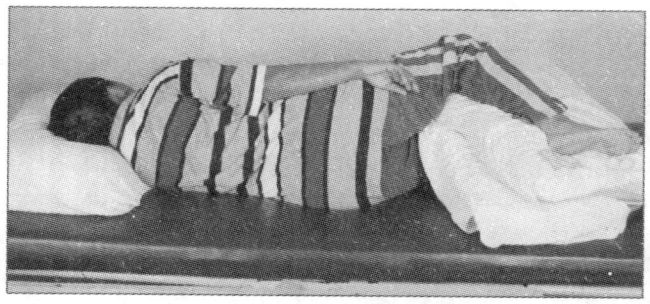

Fig. 5.6 Relaxed position – side lying (back view)

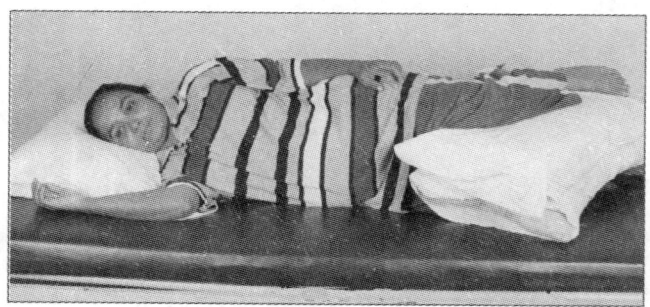

Fig. 5.7 Relaxed position – side lying (front view

c. Sitting with chair at high back rest and a towel roll on lumbar spine, the lady is completely relaxed, as seen in Fig. 5.8.

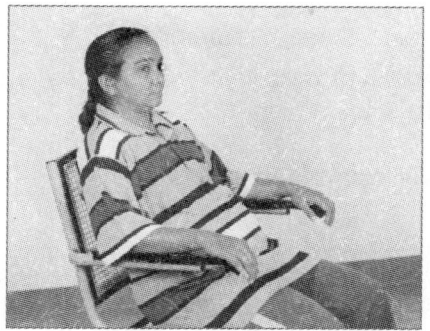

Fig. 5.8 *Relaxed sitting*

d. Sitting with head resting on a table.
There are two different ways of relaxation called as Reciprocal Relaxation and Contrast Relaxation.

Reciprocal Relaxation (Mitchel)
The antagonistic group of muscles always relax reciprocally and equally to contraction of agonist.

Sequence
Proximal to distal with commands to each part of body.
  a. To move so that tense "in folded" position -opens up.
  b. To stop moving.
  c. To let brain appreciate new posture, making patient think the new position in which body is resting.

Commands
- Take deep breath.
- Push shoulder towards feet.
- Lift arms outwards and straighten your elbows.

◎ Make whole palm of hands and fingers, fully supinated.
◎ Lower limb: Separate thighs, straighten legs, stretch feet away from the head.
◎ Press head into support of pillow.

Contrast method (Deep Breathing)
Strong contraction of muscle is followed by equal relaxation of the same muscle.

The underlying principle is:

Excitation = Inhibition

Sequence
Distal to proximal in each limb, followed by letting go on relax for an equal/longer period of time
   Then add tension in the whole limb and relaxation should be controlled in reverse sequence. For example the upper limb sequence is described below.
Upper Limb
Make a fist and let go
Tighten the wrist and let go
Tighten the elbow and let go
Tighten the shoulder and let go
Then for whole arm and let go
Similarly, for leg and head and trunk

EXERCISES

For Upper Limb Strengthening

Serratus Anterior
The lady is in supine, therapist gives her arm where lady punches through her arm with elbow straight and tries to strengthen the protractors (serratus anterior). Eventually, the same exercise is performed in sitting and in standing positions.

The Retractors

The lady is explained the action of the retractors and is asked to try to bring her shoulder blades close together; this is called *retraction*.

The lady is in high sitting position and is asked to retract and therapist gives resistance, trying to hold the medial border of the scapulae.

The lady is in standing position, an elastic band is kept at shoulder height with elbow flexed and she pulls the band towards itself retracting her shoulder blades.

Standing Push Ups

The lady performs exercises in standing, making an effort to push the wall.

(As the pregnant lady's abdomen is bulging, it becomes difficult for her to go in prone position.)

Dumb Bell Exercises

To start with the exercises:

◎ Lady will lift half a kilogram dumbbell in her hands and bend her both elbows trying to touch the shoulders. The lady is comfortable while exercising lying supine, as seen in Fig. 5.9.

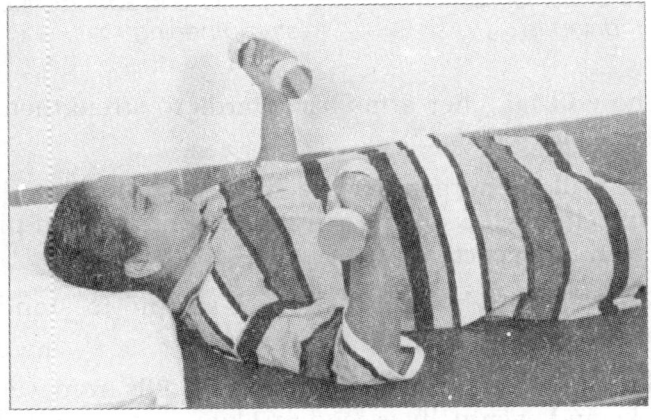

Fig. 5.9 *Biceps strengthening*

◎ She will take shoulders high up in air without bending elbows to strengthen her shoulder flexors (Fig. 5.10).

◎ She will take her arms outstretched in abduction to strengthen her abductors (Fig. 5.11).

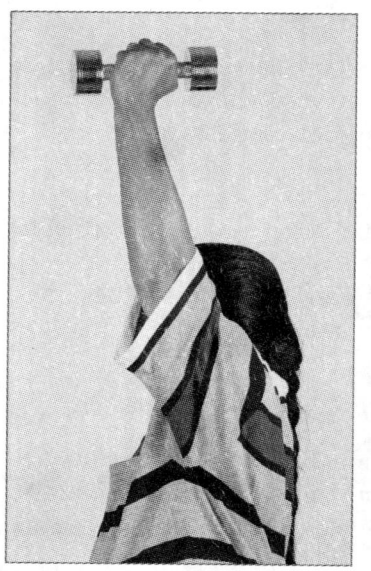 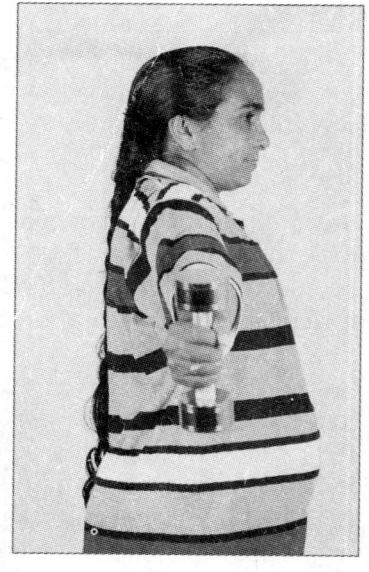

Fig. 5.10 *Shoulder flexor strengthening*

Fig. 5.11 *Shoulder abductor strengthening*

◎ She will take her arms backwards to strengthen her extensors (Fig. 5.12).

◎ She will strengthen her brachialis and brachioradialis with elbows flexed, forearm in pronation and mid-prone position respectively.

◎ She can slowly progress from supine to standing position.

◎ She can increase the weight of dumbbells from ½ kg to 1 kg and eventually ascend to 2 kg.

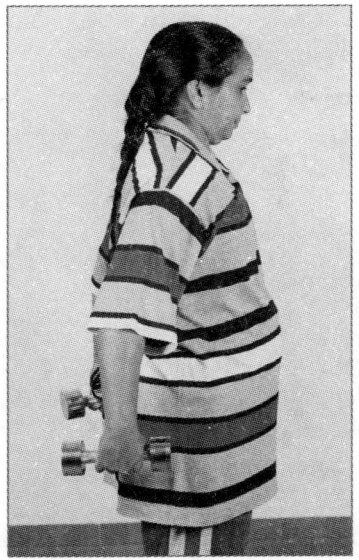

Fig. 5.12 *Shoulder extensor strengthening*

For Strengthening the Lower Limbs

◎ The lady is in supine position, she will raise her one leg without bending her knees (Fig. 5.13).

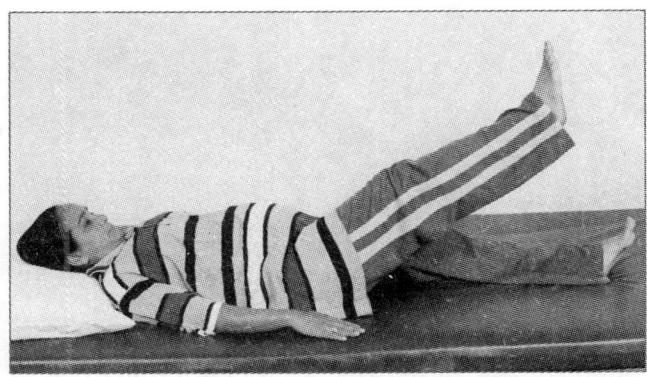

Fig. 5.13 *Straight leg raising*

◉ She will abduct her legs outwards as far as possible and bring them close (Fig. 5.14).

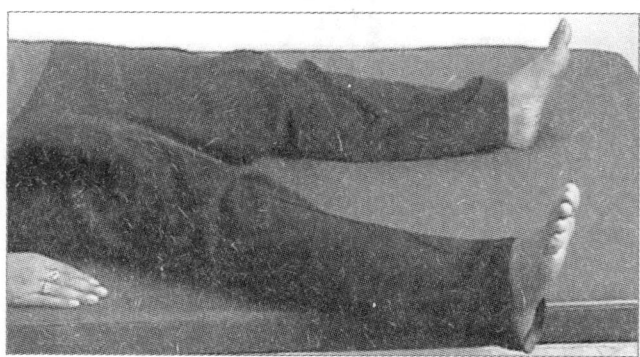

Fig. 5.14 Leg abduction

◉ *Pelvic bridging* She will raise her pelvis up in air with feet supported on couch or mat and hold it for a count of five. This action is called **pelvic bridging**. Figure 5.15 how the lady should be performing this exercise.

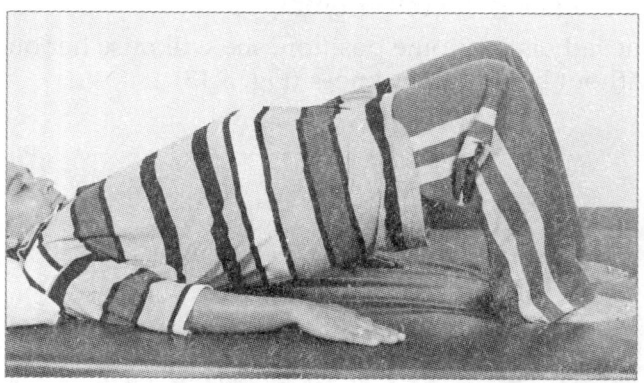

Fig. 5.15 Pelvic bridging

◉ She will go in prone position and raise her leg in the air straight for hip extensors as shown in Fig. 5.16, which she should not do after her fourth month of pregnancy.

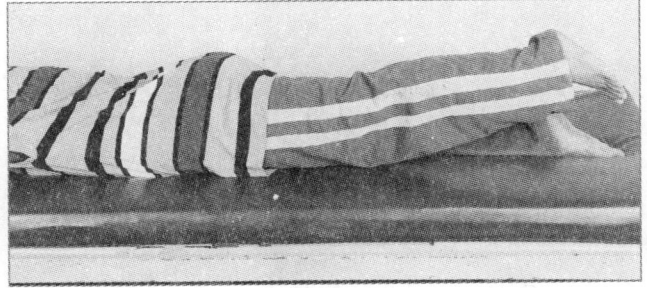

Fig. 5.16 Hip extension

◎ *Modified squatting*   The lady will hold the back rest of a chair and squat as depicted in Fig. 5.17. This strengthens hip and knee extensors and stretches the perineal area.

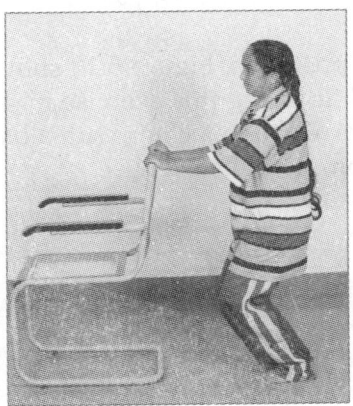

Fig. 5.17 Squatting

◎ *Wall slides*   The lady stands with her back against wall and feet at shoulder's width and slides her back down the wall as hips and knees flex (Fig. 5.18).

Stretching Exercises

◎ *Scapular protraction*   She can try to bring both scapulae borders close to each other. This can be done in sitting

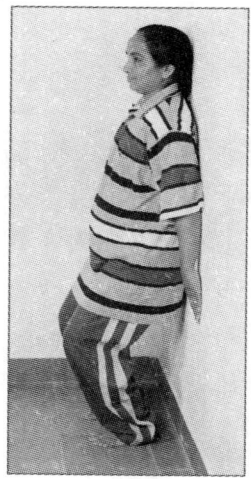

Fig. 5.18 Wall slides

or standing positions. Figure 5.19 shows it in standing position. While doing this exercise in sitting position, a stool is preferred than a chair with a back rest as it will restrict to complete the exercise.

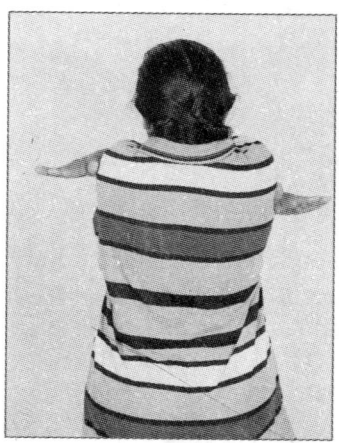

Fig. 5.19 Protraction of both scapulae

◎ *Adductor stretching* She is in sitting position where she tries to abduct her legs with knees bent and trying to touch the toes together (Fig. 5.20).

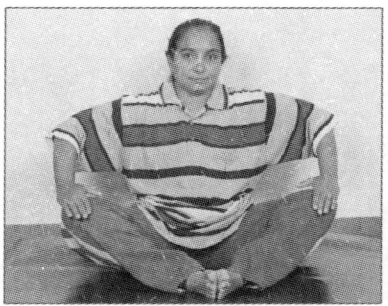

Fig. 5.20 *Adductor stretching*

◎ Sitting on a short stool, with hips abducted and feet flat on floor, adductors can be stretched.

◎ *Calf stretching* She is in lunge position where she leans forward on her bent knee, stretching the calf of opposite leg (Fig. 5.21).

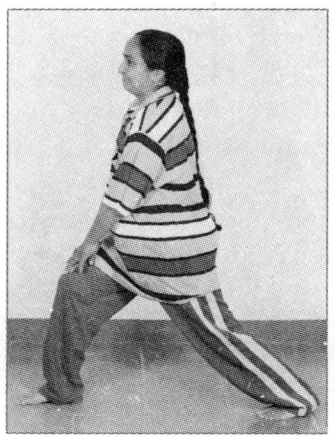

Fig. 5.21 *Left calf muscle stretching*

◎ *Pectoral stretching* She stands facing the wall and takes her arm in T-shape and V-shape to stretch her clavicular and sternal fibres respectively. In Fig. 5.22 the lady is shown doing V-shaped stretching of her pectoral muscles.

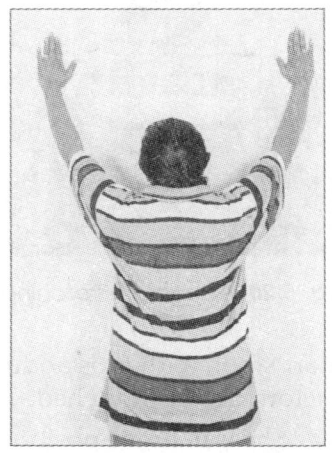

Fig. 5.22 *Pectoral muscle stretching*

◎ *Hamstrings stretching* She is in long sitting position and with the help of a towel roll tries to dorsiflex the ankles and thereby stretch hamstrings, as shown in Fig. 5.23.

◎ *Triceps and biceps* Triceps and biceps stretching is also added. Figure 5.24 shows the stretching of triceps, while Fig. 5.25 shows the stretching of biceps.

◎ *Piriformis (left)* The lady, lying in supine position, is given supine lying position with instructions to flex the hip, adduct and externally rotate with body-weight lowering towards the right side, as shown in Fig. 5.26.

Child Birth Preparation

Aims

1. To build up muscle support during pregnancy and labour.

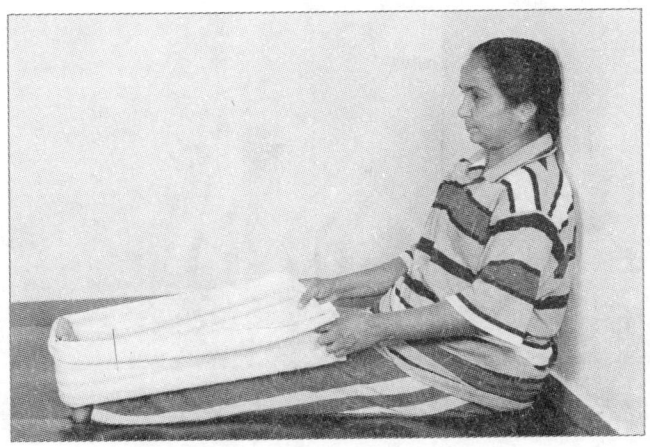

Fig. 5.23 *Auto–hamstring stretching*

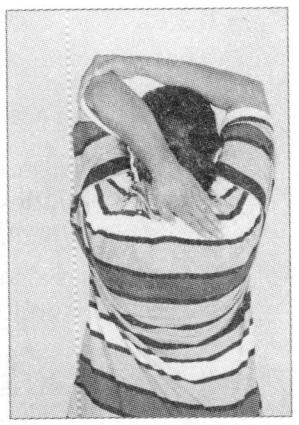

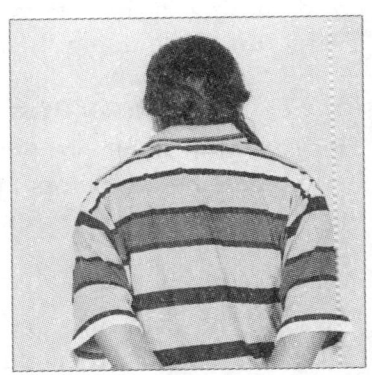

Fig. 5.24 *Triceps stretching*   **Fig. 5.25** *Biceps stretching*

2. To improve oxygenation to the tissues.
3. To enhance pushing during delivery.
4. To improve tone of the perineal muscles.

Steps to Follow

1. Exercises are done on a hard surface , i.e. a coir mattress
2. Avoid soft and sagging mattresses

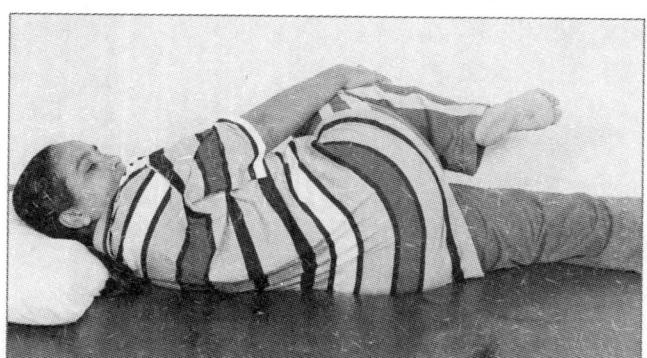

Fig. 5.26 *Right piriformis stretching*

3. All exercises are done slowly rhythmically without increasing the fatigue levels
4. Increase the repetition of exercises gradually
5. Breathing is done through nose and exhaled through mouth while doing them.

Tailor Sitting and Tailor Press

This is a comfortable position during pregnancy and labour. It stretches the adductors and helps to shift the weight of the uterus from back to front of the pelvis.

Position

The lady sits with hips and knees flexed, soles of the feet together and ankles lying parallel to each other, as shown in Fig. 5.27. In this position, she inhales deeply and while exhaling with short puffs she pushes knee towards floor.

Tailor Reach

The aim of this exercise is to improve posture, to stretch muscles of the back and to increase chest expansion. It prevents indigestion and heart burn.

The lady sits in the tailor's position where her elbows are flexed to 90 degrees. She looks up towards ceiling when she

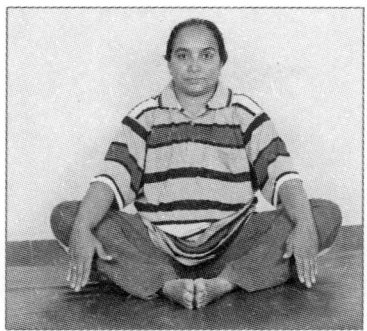

Fig. 5.27 Tailor sitting

inhales and slowly takes her one arm up in the air, while exhaling she lowers her raised arm. The same way she does with other arm and then both the arms simultaneously together (Figs 5.28 and 5.29).

Pelvic Tilts

This is a very important exercise for a pregnant lady during her gestation period and also after her delivery, i.e. postnatal period.

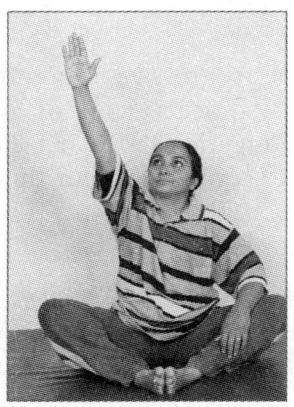

Fig. 5.28 Tailor reach

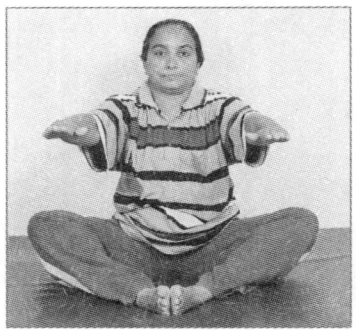

Fig. 5.29 *Tailor reach with both arms*

This is a multipurpose exercise and its purposes are to:
1. Strengthen the abdominal muscles
2. Improve posture.
3. Prevent backache.
4. Relieve back pain, if present.

There are two pelvic tilts, *anterior* and *posterior*.

The lady is told to imagine her pelvis like a trough of water supported on two vertical bars which are the legs. This trough of water stabilises by different muscle actions of hip flexors, spinal extensors and lower abdominal muscles. When this trough tilts in the forward direction, it is known as *anterior pelvic tilt* and when it tilts backward it is called as posterior pelvic tilt.

As the pregnancy progresses, it increases weight more in the abdominal area due to growing foetus and lumbar regions goes into exaggerated forward shift, i.e. an increased anterior pelvic tilt to compensate for this and to maintain a good posture she is taught pelvic tilts (posterior) in different positions like lying, sitting, standing and quadruped.

Lying supine   Lying supine with knees flexed and feet flat on the floor.

The lady is instructed to draw up and in her lower abdominal muscles and thereby flattening the lumbar curve. During this exercise she should not hold her breath. To avoid this she can count 1, 2, 3, 4, 5.

Standing   Standing with knees apart, she keeps one hand under the belly and other over sacrum (Fig. 5.30). She slowly lifts the belly and simultaneously pushes the sacrum towards the floor and is told not to hold her breath.

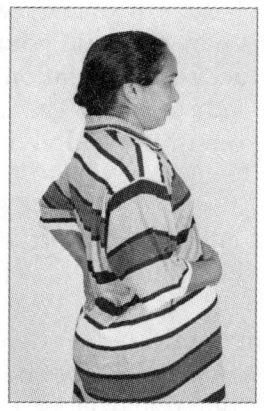

Fig. 5.30 *Pelvic tilt in standing*

Prone kneeling/quadruped/kneeling on all fours   She kneels with back straight, pulls up the abdominal muscles and tucks the belly in giving back a hunched posture (Fig. 5.31). This position is very effective as it removes the load of the uterus off the spine and out of the pelvis where it presses

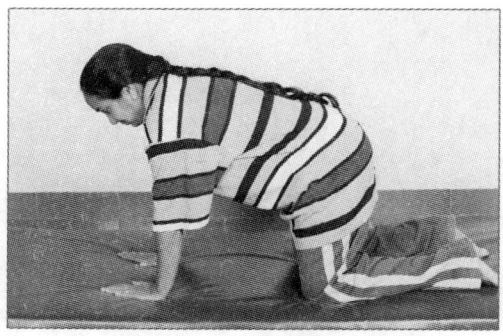

Fig. 5.31 *Prone-kneeling*

on major blood vessels. Therefore, this exercise relieves circulatory congestion, nerve twinges and pelvic pressure.

Exercises for Back Care

To strengthen the back muscles, it is a must for the therapist to teach the pregnant lady how to take care of her back. Also the therapist cautions her: "Handle your back with care"

Prone position reduces the circulation to the womb and is uncomfortable for the lady to adopt. Therefore, other positions like standing, sitting or supine/side-lying are preferred.

Exercises

  i. Static/isometric abdominal exercises are taught with a towel roll under her tummy which is shown in Fig. 5.32.
  ii. Straight peg raising.
  iii. In Fig. 5.33, simple curl ups are shown in crook-lying position where the lady touches her knees with hands.
  iv. Pelvic tilting (a dynamic exercise) should be taught in crook and side lying, sitting and standing positions.
  v. In crook-lying position, the lady crosses her hands over abdomen, fingers outside the lateral border of recti, and then oppose, with head and shoulder raise.
  vi. Oblique curl-ups are taught for obliques muscles training as shown in Fig. 5.34.

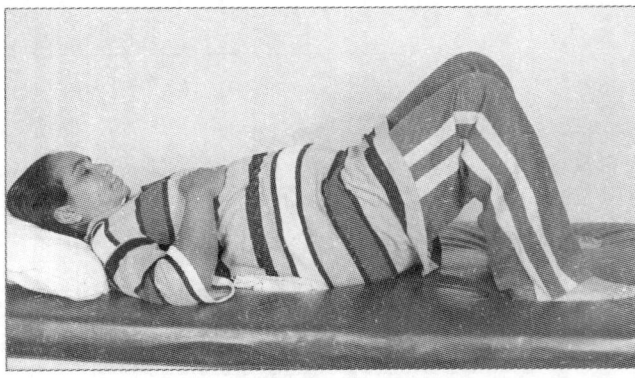

Fig. 5.32 *Static abdominals*

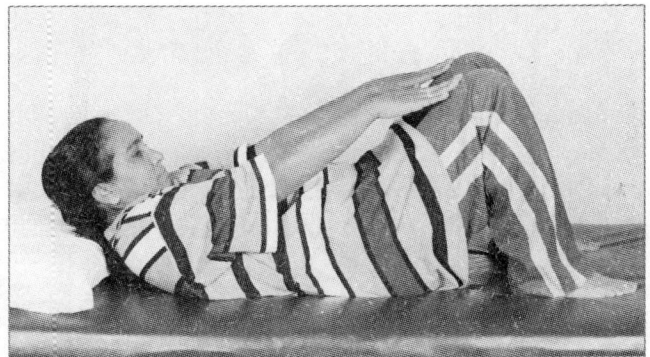

Fig. 5.33 *Curl-ups*

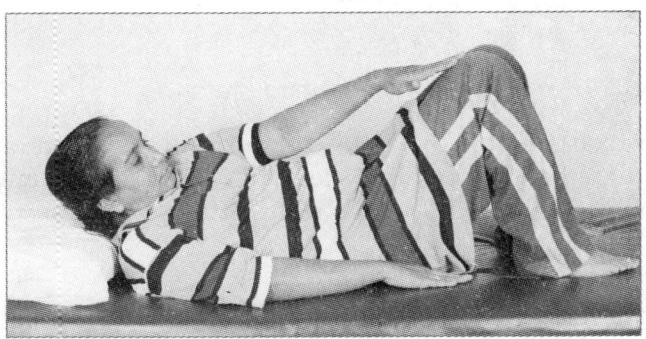

Fig. 5.34 *Oblique curl-ups with hands trying to touch the opposite knee*

Theraband Exercises

The lady sitting on chair or high stool. While using theraband, ask her to do the following.
  a. Roll the trunk to right and left alternatively.
  b. Retract her upper back using the retractors of the upper back.
  c. Rotate with extension.
  d. Patient uses thera-band under the foot opposite to the side being exercised in standing. The lady pulls against resistance extending and rotating the back (Fig. 5.35).

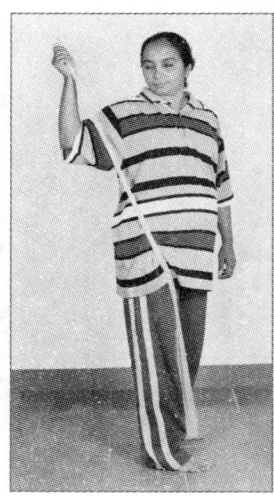

Fig. 5.35 *Thera-band stretching*

For example, for the right rotators and extensors of the back thera-band pulley is placed under the left foot, and the lady starts pulling it towards right with rotation.

Back Extensors Stabilization Exercises

On all fours or lying prone For pregnant females, all fours [quadruped/prone kneeling position is preferred than lying prone. To start with, first raises her one leg, holds for five counts and then relaxes (Fig. 5.36). In the similar manner she lifts her other leg, holds it and relaxes.

The next progressive step She lifts her one arm and contralateral leg, say she raises her right arm simultaneously raising her left leg, holds it for 5 counts and then relaxes (Fig. 5.37). In a similar fashion she does for the right leg and left arm.

Bridging Exercises

It uses co-contraction of the flexors, extensors of the trunk.

The lady is in crook lying position with hips and knees flexed; she lifts her both buttocks up from couch, holds the

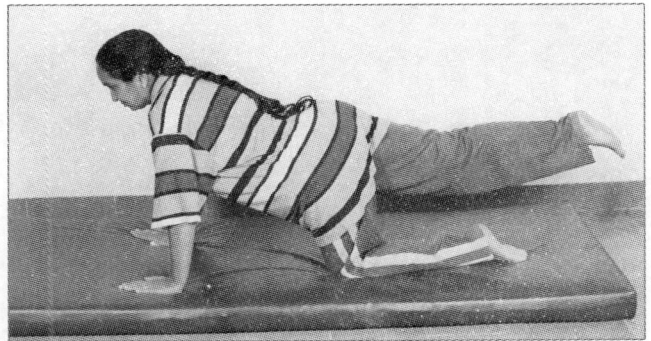

Fig. 5.36 *Prone-kneeling with one leg raised in air*

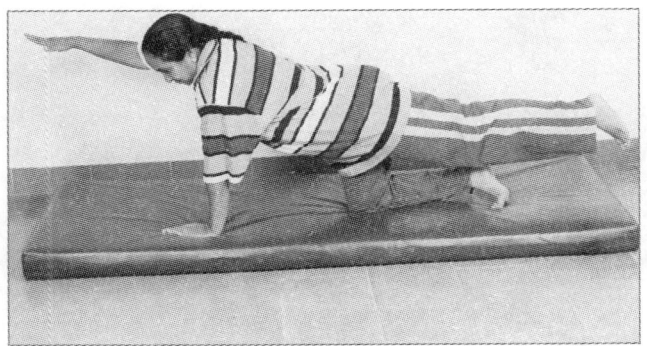

Fig. 5.37 *Prone-kneeling with right arm and left leg raised in air*

lift for 5 counts and then relaxes (Fig. 5.38). As lifting the pelvis resembles a bridge, these exercises are called *pelvic bridging exercises*.

The controlled contraction of different muscles can be strengthened by simultaneously lifting of pelvis along with one leg raised straight in air while other leg is flexed at hip and knee (Fig. 5.39). The same exercise is done with alternate lifting of the leg straight and the other leg on the couch.

Caution This exercise should not be overdone as it increases the demand by foetus from the placenta.

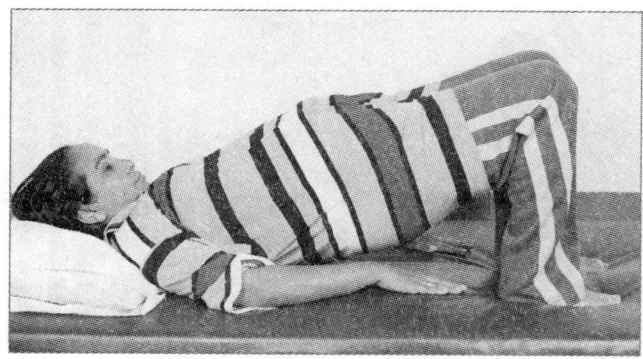

Fig. 5.38 Pelvic bridging

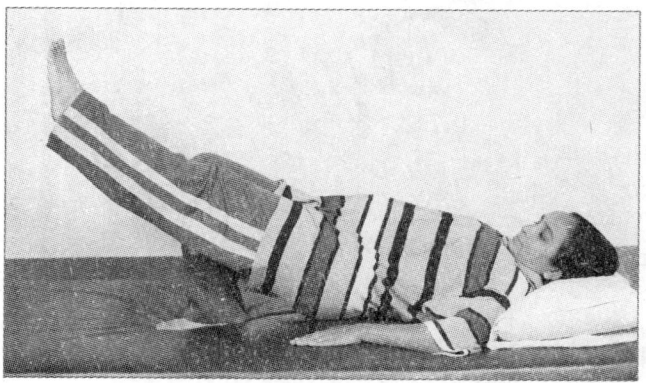

Fig. 5.39 Pelvic bridging with left leg raised in air

Straight Leg Raising

Supine lying In supine position the lady lifts her leg straight in air, holds it for five counts and then relaxes, and she does alternatively with other leg. In one session she repeats five 5 times for each leg.

Chapter 6
Pelvic Floor Exercises

THIRD SESSION

Pelvic floor training is given in third session.

Pelvic Floor Exercises

These exercises help in improving the strength of the pelvic floor muscles.

Advantages

1. Exercising the pelvic floor prenatally improves support for the uterus and other pelvic organs during pregnancy.
2. These exercises also provide greater relaxation during the pushing stage of delivery so that the muscles are more supple and controlled.
3. After the baby is born these exercises promote fast healing of the episiotomy and assist in regaining the normal strength and tone of the muscles.
4. They will also help in preventing urinary stress incontinence (an involuntary passage of urine brought on by exertion, coughing, sneezing lifting, etc.)
5. Lastly, the exercises are important throughout life for maintaining the pelvic muscles tone.

Kegel Exercises

Contraction and relaxation of the pelvic floor. As the lady very well knows the configuration and arrangement of pelvic area, it becomes easy to make her understand the exercise.

The lady imagines figure of 8 with the vaginal and urethral (urinary passages) sphincter in the front half and anal sphincter in the back half. It is the front half that needs to be strengthened. To accomplish this she is taught to constrict her muscles as if she is trying to stop her urinary flow. This is held for a count of 6 and then released. This exercise can be done in standing, sitting or lying down positions (Fig. 6.1).

Imagining Elevator/Staircase Ride

The lady is asked to imagine that she is riding in an elevator and as she ascends to each floor (beginning from the first) she is asked to draw up the perineal muscles a little more without losing any tension. When she reaches the 5th floor she holds for a few seconds and then begin to descend floor by floor again gradually relaxing the muscles in stages until she reaches the basement again.

Figure 6.2 shows how imagining an escalator/staircase ride acts as a simulator for performing pelvic floor exercises.

Mid-flow Urine Exercises

When the lady goes to the toilet, say 10 times in a day, she is advised to hold the urine in her mid-flow for 10 counts and then slowly empties her bladder. She should do this exercise only 3–4 times of her toilet visit.

Strengthening of Pelvic Floor Muscles

Once the lady has learnt to do pelvic floor exercises, she is trained for its strengthening.

◎ *Vaginal cones* These are the small weight cones, which are used for strengthening. The lady holds cones of different weights, starting from the lowest scale, in her pelvic floor area and tries to contract the muscles, so that it does not drop down. She starts this exercise in lying position, then goes for sitting position.

Eventually she walks holding the vaginal cones contracting her pelvic floor area.

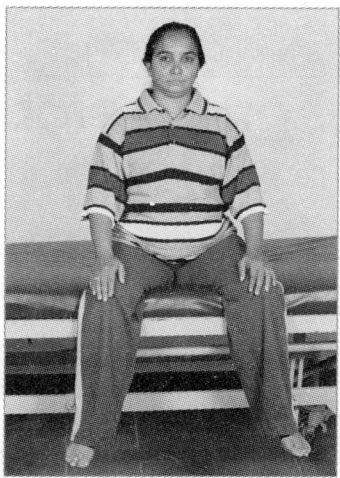

Fig. 6.1 *Kegel exercise – high sitting*

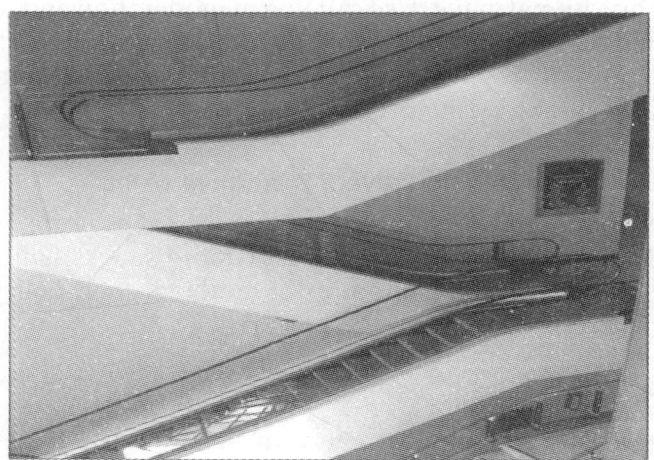

Fig. 6.2 *Escalator simulating pelvic floor exercise*

◎ As vaginal cones are expensive and not readily available, cost-effective tampoons and soft cotton balls are used to strengthen the pelvic floor muscles.

Chapter 7
Diet and Aerobics

DIET IN PREGNANCY

The lady concentrates on eating healthy, well-balanced meals without depriving or overindulging in food. She especially eats plenty of folate-rich foods such as green, leafy vegetables. Good nutrition is important for both the mother and baby. While pregnancy is not the time to start a diet, it is also not the time to eat excessively. Whether consuming regular meals or snacks, avoid foods high in calories with little nutritional value. Use caffeine in moderation and avoid drinking alcohol.

Figure 7.1 presents a diet pyramid for ideal planning of the food intake by the pregnant women.

Regular Meals Help to Prevent Premature Births

It is recommended that pregnant women should eat regular meals. Three meals a day plus 2 or more snacks is ideal. . Eating frequent, small amounts of food is a good policy for pregnant ladies.

Dietary Supplements

In general, a pregnant woman should not take any prescription or over-the-counter medications without first consulting her doctor. However, the doctor may recommend to a supplement of folic acid (500 µg) before conception until the 12th week of pregnancy. This helps in reducing the risk of brain and neural tube defects in child. If the first child has

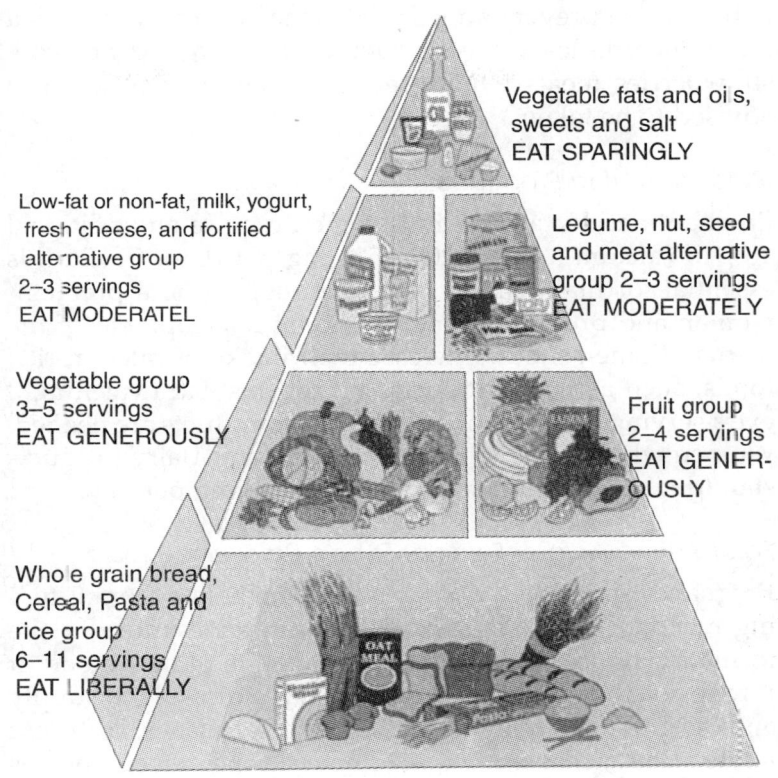

Fig. 7.1 *Diet pyramid*

been born with spina bifida or another neural tube defect, a higher-than-usual supplement of folic acid may be needed.

Diet Nutrition During Pregnancy

Dietary Advice on Vitamins, Minerals and Nutrients During Pregnancy

Iron During Pregnancy

Iron is needed in larger doses, especially in the later stages of pregnancy. This mineral is essential to the formation of healthy red blood cells. Pregnant women should eat iron-rich foods to prevent an iron deficiency-anaemia. Iron-rich foods include leafy greens such as spinach and broccoli, strawberries, meats, whole grains. Iron supplements are also advised to be taken.

Calcium During Pregnancy

Pregnant and lactating adult women require an additional 40% of calcium a day (1200–1500 mg per day). Calcium is essential for maintaining the bone integrity of a pregnant woman and providing for the skeletal development of the foetus. Women should increase their intake of calcium-rich foods, such as milk products. To get this extra calcium, 3 extra servings (3 cups) of milk or dairy products are needed. Women who do not drink milk or consume dairy products should take a calcium supplement of 600 mg per day.

Folate (Folic Acid or Folacin) During Pregnancy

Pregnancy doubles a woman's need for folate from 2 to 4 mg per day. Folate is essential for protein synthesis, the formation of new cells, and the production of new blood. It is required for a pregnant woman's expanding blood supply and the growth of both maternal and foetal tissues. Sufficient folate also decreases the risk of neural tube defects such as spina bifida.

Folate Deficiency During Pregnancy

Severe folate deficiency can result in a condition called megaloblastic anemia, which occurs most often in the last trimester of pregnancy. In this condition, the mother's heart, liver and spleen may become enlarged which can threaten the life of the foetus. Folic acid is present in many foods, including kidney beans, leafy green vegetables, peas and liver. Women in their childbearing years should consume plenty of these foods.

Folate rich food Folate-rich foods include eggs, leafy vegetables, oranges and legumes.

Vitamin D During Pregnancy

Vitamin D is necessary for the absorption of calcium and is important for normal bone growth. For women with low intake of vitamin D-fortified milk, especially those who have minimal exposure to sunlight, the daily supplementation should include 10 micrograms.

Protein During Pregnancy

The requirement for protein in pregnancy is 60 gm, which is about 15 gm more than the normal. Protein-containing foods can be excellent sources of vitamins and minerals such as iron, vitamin B_6, and zinc.

Sodium During Pregnancy

Although sodium need not be restricted during pregnancy, excessive use is not recommended. A diet of primarily natural foods can be safely salted "to taste." But women should avoid processed or "junk" foods that are high in sodium. Too much salt can lead to hypertension, and the consumption of too much salty food is related to too much weight-gain in women.

Medications

Almost any medication taken by the mother affects the baby (even something as simple as aspirin), so avoid taking any unless approved by doctor. If she suffers from a condition requiring medication, the doctor gives a drug which will not jeopardise baby.

Listeriosis

This infection is caused by a common bacterium *Listeria monocytogenes* that is present on the surface of raw, unwashed vegetables and some processed foods. Although it is rare, infection with this germ can have serious consequences for unborn babies. It can cause miscarriage, premature birth, stillbirth or result in a very sick baby.

The only way to prevent this illness is to avoid those foods in which the bacterium can live and multiply. A simple rule is to eat only foods that have been freshly cooked or prepared in the previous 12 hours. Even refrigeration does not kill the listeria bacterium.

Avoid certain foods like

◎ processed and cold meats,
◎ soft cheeses, pre-prepared salads
◎ cold, smoked or raw seafood.

Hard cheeses, fresh pasteurised milk, yoghurt, canned foods and fresh washed vegetables and fruit are safe to consume.

DIET PYRAMID

The diet pyramid, as shown in Fig. 7.1, explains the food items to be taken during the pregnancy from bulk amounts to the least in form of a pyramid. The apex of the pyramid demands to use sweets and oils or other fattening products in minimum amounts and the base asks to prefer energy giving products in large amounts.

Aerobic Exercises

Aerobic exercise is vigorous physical activity that stimulates breathing and blood circulation. For example, noncontact exercises such as swimming, static cycling. The pregnant women do aerobic exercise for up to one hour, three to four times a week to improve their physical fitness and body image.

During pregnancy, the body increases its blood volume by 40%; heart rate increases by roughly 15 beats per minute, so nutrients and oxygen can be transported to the foetus more efficiently.

◎ The respiratory rate increases, decreasing the amount of O_2 (oxygen) available for exercise so, the lady gets tired soon.

◉ The relaxin, a hormone, running through blood makes lady more flexible for exercises and delivery. With all these changes it's a good to keep doing general exercises to feel good and keep the baby safe.

Following are some of the General exercises to keep moving.

1. *Walking* Walking is always one of the best and most convenient exercises. Prefer to wear loose, light clothing (to deflect the sun), and well-supported and cushioned shoes (preferably running shoes) for walking.

2. *Swimming* Swimming is an excellent form of exercise.

Besides swimming, water walking (Fig. 7.2) and jogging are excellent forms of exercise during pregnancy.

3. *Aerobics* In low to moderate intensity aerobic exercises choreographed to music are fun, that too in a group. During these exercises, avoid any weight-lifting above the head, jumping, or lying down.

4. *Cycling on a stationary bike* This is a good weight-supporting exercise which is quite easy to perform.

Horseback riding, mountain climbing, scuba diving, skiing etc. should be avoided by pregnant women.

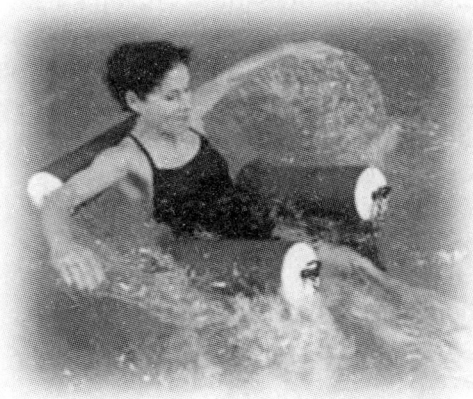

Fig. 7.2 *Water exercises*

Chapter 8
Bothering Channels

This chapter deals with the common concerns of a pregnant lady.

CARPAL TUNNEL SYNDROME

Compression of the structures of the wrist (long flexor tendons) in the confined space of the hand (carpal tunnel) which may or may not be accompanied with squeezing of the nerve which can lead to loss of sensation in the thumb zone and index and middle finger along with weakness of hand muscles.

The lady complains of pain in the wrist, which increases with repetitive activities like brushing chopping vegetables, etc.

The physiotherapist does the "Phalen's test" to elicit the symptoms of tunnel syndrome.

Phalen's test: The lady is asked to bring her plantar flexed wrists close to each other and maintain this position for 3 minutes. The complains of increased pain and disturbed sensation confirm the condition.

Physiotherapy Management
1. Resting hand splints.
2. Strengthening exercise for the upper limb.
3. Specific gripping exercises.
4. Hand care.
5. Ultrasonic therapy at the painful wrist.

RESTLESS LEG SYNDROME

Restless leg syndrome is a disorder of the nervous system with a prevalence of 5 to 10 percent in the older population. The main symptom is a distressing and almost irresistible need to move the legs, with a coexisting uncomfortable (though not usually painful) sensation deep within the legs. The sensation may be described as a muscle ache, a tension or a crawling, or feeling like ants moving in the legs or bubbles popping in the leg veins. The trouble may extend beyond the legs to involve the arms and trunk. Symptoms characteristically are brought on with rest. Movement of the legs brings relief, and avoidance of movement may promote involuntary jerks of the legs. Most often the trouble comes at night while in bed, but might be painful when resting during the day.

Although the cause of restless leg syndrome is unknown, most experts believe it is a disorder of the nervous system's control of the muscles rather then a problem with the muscles themselves. Treatment is directed at calming the overactive nervous system. Medications are prescribed by the gynaecologist.

Massage, warm baths, exercise and relaxation techniques also help.

CRAMPS

Leg cramps, another common cause of nocturnal distress, are easily distinguished from restless legs. A cramp is a sustained pain caused by involuntary contraction of a muscle, usually in the calf but sometimes in the foot. This problem occurs more often in pregnant women.

Causes
1. Overuse of a muscle.
2. Abnormal processing of essential body salts and minerals by the muscles .
3. Calcium deficiency .

4. Vascular insufficiency
5. Abnormal nerve root pressure.
6. Occasionally a prescribed medication is the cause.

Treatment

◎   Warm baths, massage and stretching exercises may help prevent nocturnal cramps if performed before retiring to bed.
◎   As the site of cramps is usually calf muscles, it is required to stretch the muscle by forced sustained dorsiflexion or vigorous ankle and foot exercises.
◎   Deep kneading is given as a part of soft tissue mobilization.
◎   Pre-bed time walk makes a considerable difference on the following day.

The disruption of sleep caused by restless leg syndrome or nocturnal leg cramps can lead to daytime fatigue or sleepiness, alteration in mood and even confusion. Proper diagnosis and treatment is must if symptoms are frequent or severe.

MERALGIA PARAESTHETICA

This is the term given to the disorder where there is entrapment of the lateral cutaneous nerve of the thigh.

Anatomy

The lateral cutaneous nerve of the thigh emerges from the lateral border of the psoas major muscle, migrates through the pelvis and exits to become superficial approximately 1 cm medial to the anterior superior iliac spine (ASIS), underneath the inguinal ligament. The nerve then enters the fascia lata and divides into anterior and posterior divisions. Under the inguinal ligament, the nerve is relatively fixed within the fascial tissues.

Predisposing Factors

It is usually seen by six months of gestation. Predisposing factors may include the following.

◎ Obesity
◎ Flat (pronated) feet
◎ Spondylitis
◎ Tight fascia lata
◎ Post abdominal surgery (scar entrapment)
◎ Tight fitting garments, e.g. corsets or girdles

Symptoms

1. Because the nerve is cutaneous, the symptoms associated are normally paraethesias, burning sensations or occasionally pain. These symptoms are usually situated over the anterior or anterolateral surface of the thigh, in the distribution of the lateral cutaneous nerve of the thigh.
2. The most common complaints are that of symptoms on standing and/or walking/hip extension aggravating the condition. On the other hand activities that promote hip flexion, e.g. sitting will ease the symptoms.
3. Sensory loss of light touch or pin-prick.

Differential Diagnosis

Numerous other structures may refer into the area of symptoms. These may include the following.
◎ Hip joint
◎ Femoral nerve
◎ Upper lumbar spine

Treatment

Pregnant ladies who suffer from meralgia Paraesthetica are usually left untreated. They may, with time, resolve without treatment, although some form of therapeutic advice should be given. Treatments that are often performed include the following.
◎ Stretching tight fascia lata
◎ Massage and pain relieving modalities like TENS
◎ Orthotic correction
◎ Lumbar mobilization

- ◎ Neural stretching techniques (prone knee bend with hip extension and slight adduction)
- ◎ Cortisone injection
- ◎ Surgery to decompress the nerve

THE PRENATAL PAIN OF PREGNANCY

Back Pain

As the baby grows, much of this weight is carried in the front; consequently, the lady has to adjust her posture by shifting her weight back to compensate, as seen in Fig. 8.1. This change in posture puts more weight on the spinal joints which produces a tender and sore back and tight muscles. One of the most interesting changes during pregnancy is the presence of a hormone called *relaxin*. Relaxin increases 10-fold during pregnancy, reaching a maximum at 38–42 weeks. This ovarian hormone, as its name implies, is responsible for relaxing the ligaments of the pelvis in preparation for birth.

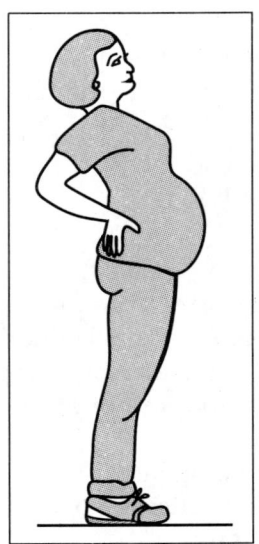

Fig. 8.1 *Bad posture—triggering back pain*

The ligaments of the pelvis are located in the sacroiliac joints and the symphysis pubis, at the front of the pelvis. The ligaments during pregnancy, brings changes in weight-shifts, LOG deviation at pelvis and vertebral column.

The pain in the back is very common complain, which is seen usually during antenatal as well as postnatal period. The pain can be at the following areas.

1. Cervical
2. Thoracic
3. Lumbar
4. Lumbosacral

Relaxin relaxes the ligaments and its levels return to normal within 3–4 days postpartum but its effects are long-lasting.

Causes of Back-Pain

1. Altered physiological and biochemical state during pregnancy.
2. Trauma during labour and delivery
3. Bad postural habits during pregnancy and postpartum.
4. Referred pain due to urinary tract infection.

Epidural Site Pain

Local pain over epidural site can be felt. This could be due to haematoma in dura and epidural space over the area of supraspinous ligament.

Management

Hot packs/ heating pad.
Ice packs.

Thoracic Pain

Pain in thoracic region are often felt due to unsupported upper back during second stage of labour and/or wrong feeding position. Therefore correct positions need to be taught, i.e. supportive back with pillows in lap and baby well supported.

Hot packs to relieve pain

Exercises

Shoulder bracing and retraction exercises.

Elbow exercises

Pelvic tilting exercises.

Note: In antenatal and postnatal classes, posture correction needs to be stressed.

Low Back Pain

Very common pain during and postpregnancy. To suppress acute pain, pain relieving modalities like hot packs and TENS are used.

For Back Pain

To strengthen the back muscles:

It is a must for the therapist to teach the pregnant lady to take care of her back. Also the therapist tells "Handle your back with care".

As the prone position is difficult for the lady to go into, the exercises are preferred in standing, sitting or supine lying.

The lady is in supine lying position: Ask her to flatten the nape of her back on the couch with neck and sacrum-isometric spinal extensor.

a. Straight leg raising: The lady lifts her leg up in the air without bending her knees, as seen in Fig. 8.2. This exercise has already been explained in Chapter 5.

b. Trunk rolling

c. Rotation with extension

d. Back extensors stabilization exercises

e. Bridging exercises

The controlled contraction of different muscles can be strengthened by simultaneously lifting of pelvis along with one leg raised straight in air while other leg is flexed at hip and knee. The same exercise is done with alternate lifting of the leg straight and the other leg on the couch.

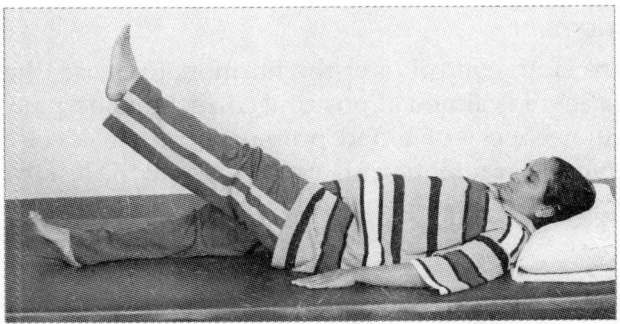

Fig. 8.2 *Straight leg raising*

Caution: The pregnant lady should not overdo this exercise as it increases the demand by foetus from placenta.

Posture care and Ergonomics
◎ Sit and stand tall.
◎ Maintain the aligned posture.
◎ Use high back rest chairs and well supported arm rests.
◎ Avoid foam mattresses
◎ Avoid high heels
◎ Avoid stoop squatting.
◎ Avoid lifting heavy weights.

Coccydynia

Pain in tail bone, i.e. coccyx and surrounding area is termed as coccydynia. This condition is seen five times more in women than men.

Causes During Pregnancy
These are
1. Hormonal changes leading to ligaments laxity which eventually puts unwanted traction on coccyx, causing strain and pain.
2. Prolonged and/or faulty postural habits.

Management

As there is no control over the hormonal release, therefore the treatment is aimed at postural correction and pain relief.

Regular checks of blood pressure, protein levels in the urine and water retention are necessary into the last trimester of pregnancy to prevent preeclampsia

PREECLAMPSIA

Up to 1 in 10 pregnant women develops raised blood pressure accompanied by the appearance of protein in the urine (proteinuria) and retention of excessive amounts of fluid in the body (oedema). It is not usually seen before the sixth month of pregnancy and most women develop the condition at the end of their pregnancy. However, only 1 out of 100 women will have the severe form of the condition. Preeclampsia can also occur up to a week following the delivery of the baby.

Aetiology

It is still not known why certain women develop high blood pressure during pregnancy.

Certain preexisting conditions increase the risk of developing high blood pressure. The include the following.

◎ First pregnancy
◎ Diabetes
◎ Essential hypertension (high pressure before pregnancy)
◎ Chronic kidney diseases
◎ Previous pregnancies affected by preeclampsia
◎ Carrying twins or triplets

Symptoms

◎ Hypertension (high blood pressure). As a general rule a blood pressure greater than 140/90 mm Hg in pregnancy is considered to be raised. Very high blood pressure (great than 170/110 mm Hg), often accompanied by headache and the appearance of flashing lights before the eyes. Measuring a woman's blood pressure is an essential part of any antenatal clinic visit.

◎ Protein in the urine This is detected by using a special stick to dip into a clean sample of urine. There are other causes of proteinuria but preeclampsia is the cause with most significance for the mother and foetus.

◎ Sudden or insidious weight gain with swollen hands, feet or other parts of the body. Some swelling is normal in pregnancy but it should prompt a woman to have her blood pressure and urine checked.

◎ Pain in the right upper abdomen may indicate involvement of liver which in severe cases can be complicated by an imbalance of the coagulation system that causes an increased or decreased ability of the blood to clot.

◎ Headache, fatigue and pains in the upper abdomen

These are all symptoms of the more severe stage of the condition.

Preeclampsia is often subdivided into mild, moderate and severe varieties, depending on the level of blood pressure and the involvement of other organs in the disease process. In the worst cases, preeclampsia can develop into eclampsia, a situation where the mother has a convulsion. Fortunately, eclampsia is rare, but this is largely because women with preeclampsia are usually detected and treated before eclampsia can develop.

All the symptoms will disappear after the delivery and normally the blood pressure and protein level in the urine will be back to normal after a maximum of two weeks.

Treatment

The primary aim is to monitor the mother and the foetus closely. This may require hospital admission. Preeclampsia can, in severe cases, influence the placental function and diminish the flow of nourishment and oxygen to the foetus, which will slow its growth. Antihypertensive medicines of different groups are often used to reduce blood pressure.

If the woman's condition deteriorates and the foetus is at risk, the only solution is to deliver the baby either by induction of labour or by performing a caesarean section.

Prevention

Monitoring of the woman's blood pressure and urine is essential. If hypertension is developing, it is vital to measure the blood pressure and test urine for protein regularly.

PREGNANCY DIABETES/GESTATIONAL DIABETES

Diabetes is a condition where the blood glucose (sugar) level is higher than normal.

Types of Diabetes

There are two major forms of diabetes:

◎ Type 1 diabetes, or *insulin-dependent diabetes*. This type is often seen in young people.

◎ Type 2 diabetes, or *non insulin-dependent diabetes*. This type tends to affect the elderly or overweight people.

Other types include:

◎ *Gestational diabetes*. This type is often associated with pregnancy and usually disappears after birth.

◎ *Secondary diabetes*. This usually occurs as the result of some other condition in the body such as inflammation of the pancreas, or the use of certain medications such as steroids or diuretics.

Type 1 Diabetes (Diabetes Mellitus)

Thus is a long-term disease of the pancreas gland, which is situated within the abdomen. Every cell in the body needs insulin (a hormone released in response to increased levels of sugar in the blood) in order for glucose (blood sugar) to be absorbed into the body's cells. If the body is deficient in insulin, then glucose will build up in the bloodstream. Type 1 diabetes can appear at any age. Every patient affected needs insulin injections to avoid the complications of insulin deficiency.

When the glucose level gets sufficiently high, it starts showing up in the urine.

Type 2 Diabetes

This is also known as non-insulin dependent diabetes. Every cell in the body needs insulin to absorb glucose (sugar) from the bloodstream. In Type 2 diabetes the pancreas does not make sufficient insulin to overcome the resistance to insulin seen in this type of diabetes. When the glucose level gets sufficiently high, glucose will appear in the urine.

Type 2 diabetes is most common in overweight adults. Insulin injections are not always needed since proper dieting or tablets can usually control it, especially in the first five years after diagnosis.

Aetiology

The hormone insulin is produced in the pancreas and acts to decrease blood sugar. During pregnancy women require more insulin, and diabetes occurs if the body is not able to produce the increased amounts. After delivery, the need for insulin decreases back to normal level where the diabetes will disappear. A mother who has had pregnancy diabetes will have an increased risk of developing Type 2 diabetes later on in life as the production of insulin decreases with increasing age. This risk can be considerably reduced if a healthy lifestyle is adopted. This should involve a healthy diet, followed by regular exercise and maintaining a healthy body weight.

Symptoms

In most cases, pregnancy diabetes shows no external symptoms and is detected through screening. Only rarely do symptoms appear.

Screening can be done in the following ways.

A pregnant woman will have her fasting blood sugar measured. This is done if she has one or more of the following characteristics.

◎ A family history of Type 1 or Type 2 diabetes
◎ History of birth of very large children (over 4 kg)
◎ Overweight prior to pregnancy
◎ Pregnancy at or above 35 years of age
◎ Glucose is present in the urine.

If the fasting person's blood glucose value is in 'grey zone', another test is often carried out, which is called the 'sugar-loading' test. This test is able to detect the existence of pregnancy diabetes. If the blood glucose value is normal, then another reading of the blood glucose level is taken in the 32nd to 33rd week of pregnancy.

Treatment

◎ Pregnancy diabetes is always treated with a strict diabetic diet.
◎ Sometimes it is also necessary to include insulin in the treatment. Quick-acting insulin will be given at mealtimes and slow-acting insulin at bedtime.

Medication

◎ Quick-acting insulin as injection.
◎ Slow-acting insulin as injection.
◎ Mixed-insulin as injection.
◎ Note: antidiabetic tablets should be avoided because diabetes can be controlled more tightly during pregnancy with insulin and this reduces the chances of complications.

Tips

◎ Maintain a healthy 'diabetes' diet that is low in fat and rich in complex carbohydrates such as potatoes, rice and pasta. The diet should also include daily portions of fresh vegetables and fibre.

◎ The lady should measure blood sugar very regularly in order to decide if the prescribed treatment is helping.

◎ Be in touch with diabetologist, preferably in a joint clinic with a specialist obstetrician to monitor the diabetes and the baby's progress carefully during pregnancy.

◎ After the pregnancy, it is important to get examined once in a year to find out if the diabetes has developed again.

The likelihood of developing diabetes later in life can be reduced by the following:

◎ Avoiding overweight

◎ Eating a healthy diet

◎ Exercising regularly

◎ Avoiding smoking (this will benefit both the baby and mother)

Chapter 9

Stages of Labour

In labour the foetal head descends down by exerting pressure on the perineum, dilating the cervix, vagina, displacing the levator ani muscles sideways and downwards. The constant stretching and lengthening during end of first stage and beginning of second stage causes thinning of posterior portion of pelvic floor and perineum. This forms the birth canal making vaginal opening directed more anteriorly. To accelerate this delivery process, episiotomy is done. Fascia gets overstretched, muscle fibres are torn by the end of labour.

STAGES OF LABOUR: FOURTH (LAMAZE) SESSION

Figure 9.1 demonstrates the position of foetus over the abdomen (a) and in utero (b).

First stage

◎ *Prodromal:* Not everyone has this stage, but it is fairly common, can last a few days, contractions come and go and never get stronger, longer and closer together. Figure 9.2 shows the uterine contractions.

◎ *Early or latent:* Is up to 3–4 cm, and can last anywhere from 20 minutes to 20 hours.

Active: Is up to 7–8 cm and can last anywhere from 20 minutes to many hours, but is usually shorter than latent (Fig. 9.3 b).

Normal anatomy at full term (40 week)

Placenta

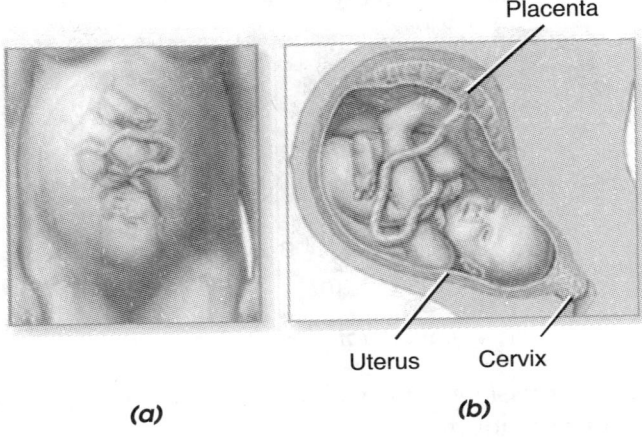

Uterus   Cervix

(a)   *(b)*

Fig. 9.1 *Demonstrating the position of fetus over the abdomen (a) and in-utero (b).*

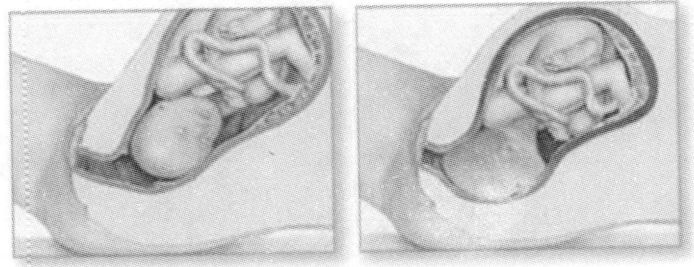

Uterus between contraction   Uterus during contraction

Fig. 9.2 *Uterine contractions*

Transition: Cervix up to 10 cm or completely gets dilated, lasts the shortest and is the most intense (Fig. 9.3c).

Second stage

◎ *Early or resting phase:* It is sometimes accompanied by an urge to push, sometimes not, can last up to 4 hours if only it was allowed.

| Undilated uneffaced | Partly dilated partly effaced | Fully dilated fully effaced |

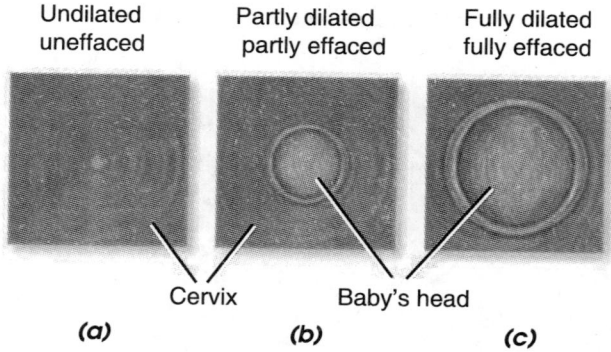

Cervix   Baby's head

(a)   *(b)*   *(c)*

Fig. 9.3 *Dilatation of cervix*

◎ *Active or pushing:* Irresistible urge to push usually lasts about two hours.

◎ *Crowning:* When baby's head is being born, as shown in Fig. 9.4. The doctor separates the new born from the mother by clamping and cutting the umbilical cord, as seen in Fig. 9.5.

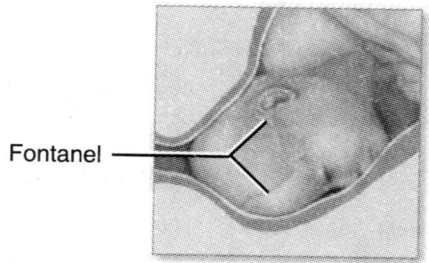

Fontanel

Fig. 9.4 *Foetal fontanels*

Third stage

◎ *Delivery of the placenta* It can take anywhere from 5 minutes to an hour or so, as depicted in Fig. 9.6.

For First Stage of Labour

Figure 9.7 shows the position of the foetus in first stage of labour.

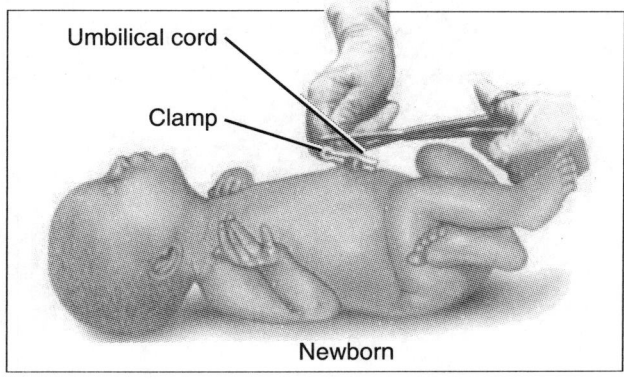

Umbilical cord

Clamp

Newborn

Fig. 9.5 *Newborn baby*

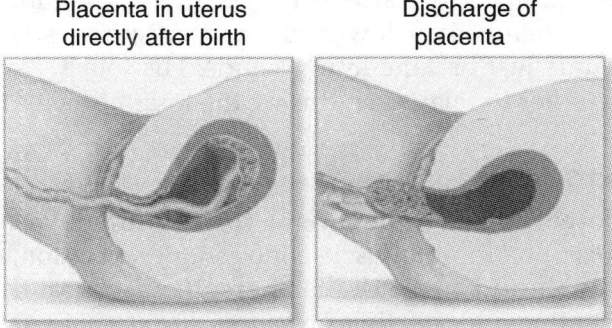

Placenta in uterus
directly after birth

Discharge of
placenta

Fig. 9.6 *Placenta discharge*

1. The lady should keep a balance of rest and gentle activity, physical and mental well being.
2. Brief periods of walking, chair/bean bags sittings, intermittent with periods of rest.
3. She is advised to empty bladder every 2 hours as a full bladder can increase pain and delay progress.

She should be taught to breathe out slowly and easily, and with it try to release the body. Let the breath – "let-go". The would-be-father can be a real asset to a would-be-mother

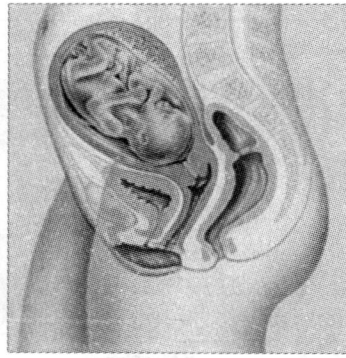

Fig. 9.7 *Foetus position in first stage of labor*

by cooperating and learning the breathing techniques. He keeps his hands over lower ribs and encourages her with command "just breathe in my hands. His touch, his voice, enhances her to relax even during the tough time of labour.

Second Stage of Labour

◎ Mother needs to be taught the rhythmicity between push, breathing, muscle contraction, relaxation, etc.

◎ She should not exhaust herself with unnecessary straining and exerting pressures.

◎ For a smooth descent, pressure needs to be exerted from above the fundus while pelvic floor muscles relax completely.

Vocalization

Her expression of pain through moans or groans not only give an insight to her needs, but also stimulate endorphins to block pain pathways.

Breathing and Pushing: Instructions

1. Keep the index finger over epigastrium, take a breathe in and feel expansion in this area.

2. Fix the ribs and increase the intrathoracic pressure. With this inspiration, bear down and the diaphragm will act as piston downwards towards fundus.
3. Place the other hand on waist, feel it expand sideways and become aware of release of her abdominal and relaxation of pelvic floor muscles.
4. Hold breath only for short periods 16–18 counts to minimize any adverse effect on foetus due to prolonged pushing maneuver.
5. Release the breath and repeat pushing techniques, take several pushes during a contraction.
6. Between the contractions, sight out, rest and relax.

Panting is practised in the last stage, when urge to push has become uncontrollable.

POSITIONING IN LABOUR

Positional change has a positive effect on the efficiency of uterine contractions.

Position in First Stage of Labour

She should be upright mobile and active in first stage of labour.

Since supine position leads to supine hypotension syndrome, this position should be avoided.

Avoid Supine Position for Labour and Delivery: Anteversion of uterus occurs during first stage of labour. Therefore, lean forward on some support. Or change of position from one to other stimulates the efficient uterine activity.

Positions preferred in this stage are as follows.
1. Relaxed half lying position as shown in Fig 9.8.
2. Kneel-sitting with head and arms resting on seat of chair (Fig. 9.9).
3. Half kneeling with arms and head resting on back rest of chair (Fig. 9.10).

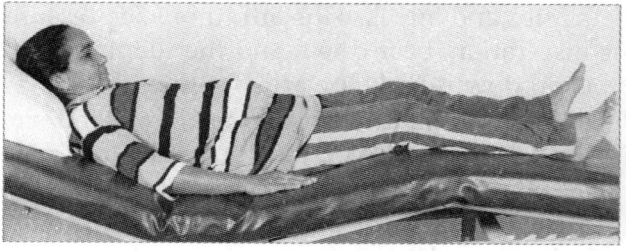

Fig. 9.8 Relaxed half lying

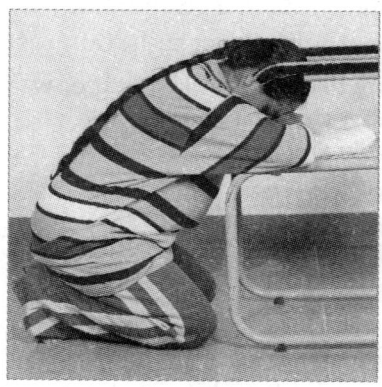

Fig. 9.9 Kneel sitting with arms and head resting in front of chair

4. Leaning on wall (Fig. 9.11).
5. Leaning forward on partner's shoulder.
6. Half-Kneeling on chair, with forward lean on partners shoulder
7. Sitting on beanbag with legs abducted.
8. Prone kneeling (quadripod, on all fours).
9. Long-sitting with pillows supporting back and under knees

Position in Second Stage

1. Side lying with one leg abducted, held in position by one hand or pillows, as seen in Fig. 9.12.

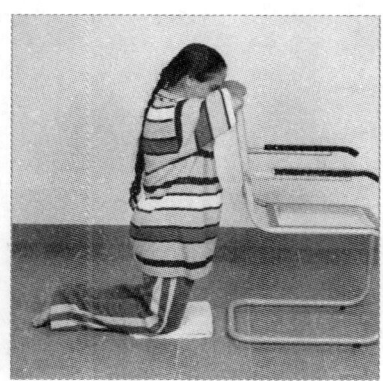

Fig. 9.10 Half kneeling with arms and head resting at backrest of chair

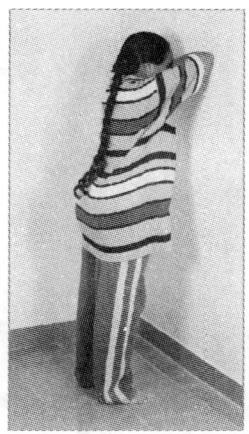

Fig. 9.11 Leaning on wall

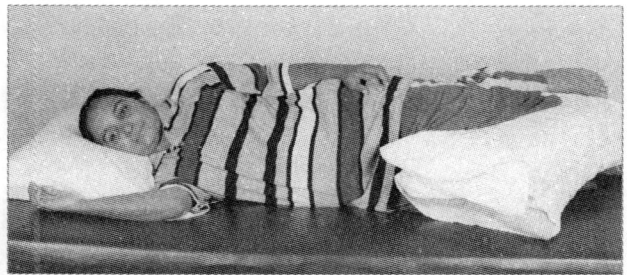

Fig. 9.12 Relaxed position – side lying

2. Crook-sitting with legs wide abducted.
3. Prone kneeling.
4. Squatting with abducted legs (Fig. 9.13).
5. Semi squats / half squats: Sitting, standing, kneeling or squatting (Fig. 9.14) are preferred more than supine and side-lying because of the following reasons.

Benefits

1. The gravitational effect of gravity can be used.

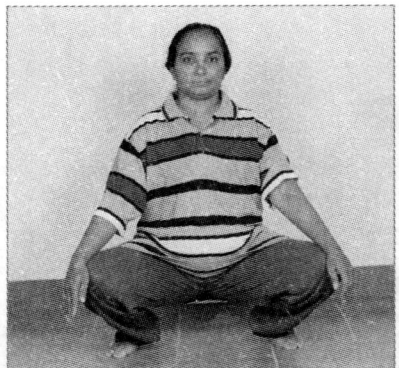

Fig. 9.13 *Squatting with legs abducted*

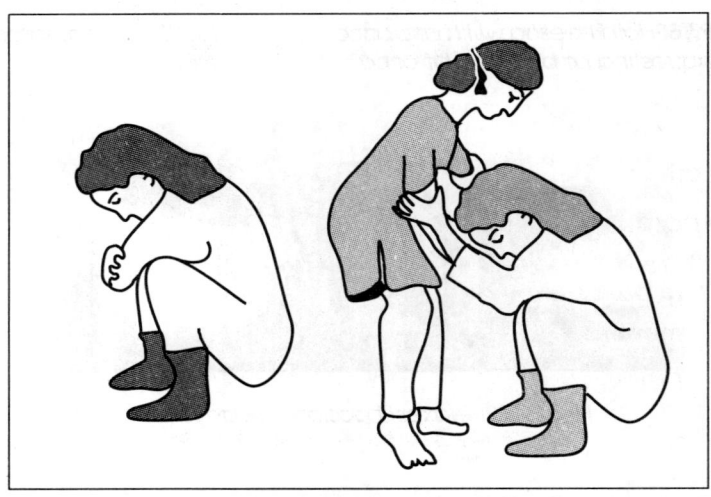

Fig. 9.14 *Encouraging squatting*

2. The pelvic outlet is more in squatting.
3. Stronger and effective contractions can be performed

Position in Third Stage

As there is risk of haemorrhage the lady is taught about its management. She is explained in detail about the procedure of expulsion of fetal head as shown in Fig. 9.15. She is also

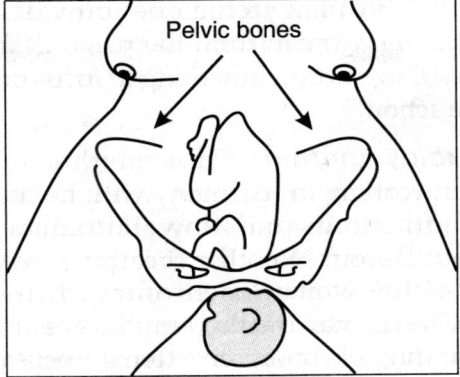

Fig. 9.15 *Expulsion of foetal head*

taught about episiotomy which is preferably a medio-lateral incision given on the vaginal surface. This prevents tears and reduces the pelvic injury.

Breathing Techniques for First Stage of Labour

Purpose of Breathing Techniques

◎ *Providing oxygen*   Provide oxygen to mother and baby. If the muscles are well-oxygenated, they can function more effectively, with less pain.

◎ *Relaxation*   Relaxation is important because pain impulses are perceived more quickly when anxiety is present; anxiety and tension also increase the body's production of adrenaline. Adrenaline causes blood vessels to constrict, reducing oxygen supply to the muscles which causes pain and decreases the production of oxytocin, thus slowing the process of labour. To prevent this vicious cycle, relaxation is taught in different ways.

◎ *Rhythmic breathing*   It promotes physical relaxation by reducing muscle tension and promotes emotional relaxation by reducing anxiety.

◎ *Distraction* Breathing techniques provide a means for distracting the woman from the pain of labour, giving her "something to do, something to focus on, other than the contraction."

◎ *The Bradley method* This method emphasizes relaxation working in harmony with the body, 'tuning in' to contractions and slow abdominal breathing throughout labour. No other breathing techniques are taught, as the woman is encouraged to follow her instincts. The Lamaze method emphasizes an intellectual understanding of labour, an external focus of attention, and distraction with patterned breathing techniques. This style is appropriate for women and couples who need a sense of being in control and is very comfortable for them.

The Cleansing Breath

◎ *How to* At the beginning of each contraction ask the lady to take a deep breath in through nose, bringing in new energy for the contraction, then exhale it through the mouth, releasing tension, sighing on the exhale, if desired. When a contraction ends, another deep cleansing breath is taken and mother is asked to relax.

◎ *When to use* No special breathing techniques are necessary in early labour, start with the breathing techniques when mother can no longer walk and talk during contraction and no longer want to be distracted between contractions.

◎ *Benefits* Welcoming breath gives both mother and baby an extra boost of oxygen, serves as a signal to relax and focus, and informs the partner and support people that a contraction has begun. Closing breath serves as a release and as a sign to inform support people and partner that contraction has passed and serves as a reminder to relax between contractions.

Slow, Relaxed, Abdominal Breathing

◎ *How to* The lady is instructed to inhale through nose allowing belly to expand first, then chest. Exhale slowly through mouth, pursing the lips to prevent mouth dryness, as shown in Fig. 9.16.

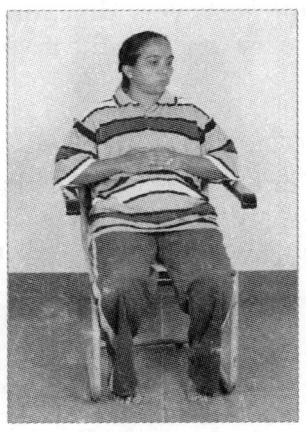

Fig. 9.16 *Slow – Relaxed abdominal breathing (sitting posture)*

◎ *Frequency* Slow and relaxed, about half the normal rate, 6–9 breaths per minute.

◎ *When to use* Women can use this breathing method throughout the entire labour. Some women find that at some point in labour, they get tense and can no longer relax with this technique, and use other breathing techniques.

◎ *Benefits* Relaxing, slow and effortless. This breathing slowly induces a sense of peacefulness and safety that helps to release tension.

Practising Before Labour

This breathing can be practised at any time While driving, reading or watching TV, at work.

◎ If the lady begins to feel light-headed or dizzy, ask her to take a deep cleansing breath, and start over again. If necessary, re-breathe the air by cupping the hands over nose and mouth, or breathing into a paper bag.

◎ This can be practised in various positions like sitting, side-lying, standing.

Tips If her mouth feels very dry during this breathing, she is encouraged to try touching the tip of the tongue to the roof of the mouth.

Hee-Hee Blow Breathing

◎ *How to* Similar to Hee-Hee breathing, except that 1 to 5 "hee" breaths are followed by a blow. The blow is a deeper, slightly slower breath and induces relaxation (Fig. 9.17).

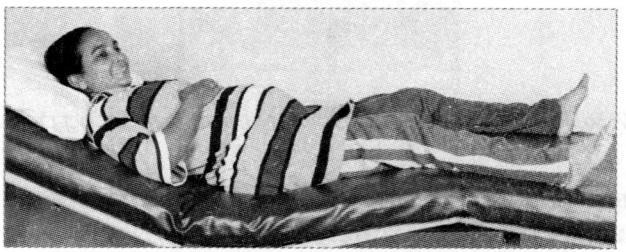

Fig. 9.17 *Hee–Hee Breathing*

◎ As always hee-hee blow breathing begins and end with a contraction with a cleansing breath.

◎ *When to use* When Hee-Hee breathing is not enough. It is helpful during transition.

◎ *Benefits of patterned hee-hee-blow* Provides a rhythm to breathing. It helps in avoiding hyperventilation. The blow breath helps to release tension.

Some women nod their heads in rhythm to the 'beat' of this breathing.

◎ *Practising* Varies with individual to individual, some women do three 'hees" with every contraction, others find more or less "hees" to be most helpful.

Variable Hee-Blow Breathing

◎ *How to* Partner randomly chooses a number of breaths to be done by the expected mom before each blow: 2, 3, or 4. For example, he holds up two fingers. If she does not like watching his fingers, he can also say a number or hold the fingers on her arm where she can feel them but does not need to look at them.

◎ *When to use* Best as a "take-charge" routine during transition. The partner can use when the women is feeling out of control and panicky. He should establish eye contact with her, and guide her through breathing until she is focused again.

◎ *Benefits* Distraction: The woman focuses on partner and on counting the breaths.

◎ *Practising* Practice with partner is the best.

Combining Techniques

The lady should always use the most basic technique possible, using the least effort required to manage each contraction. This will help in preventing fatigue. Use slow, relaxed breathing whenever possible.

Use slower, more relaxed breathing at the beginning and end of contraction.

When the contraction begins, she is instructed to do a deep, cleaning breath, switching to hee-hee breathing/hee-hee blow over the peak of the contraction returning to slow, deep breathing and with the cleansing breath at the end of the contraction.

Breathing Techniques for Second–Stage Labour

How to Avoid Pushing, if Necessary

1. *How to* She lifts the chin and arches the back a little. Either breathe deeply relaxing the body or pant blowing lightly. She can imagine or visualize a feather and blow just enough to keep the feather bouncing up and down in the air above lips.

2. *When to use* If she is experiencing the urge to push, and the caregiver feels that it is too early to begin pushing or that there is some need to stop pushing temporarily.

3. *Benefits* This breathing will not prevent the uterus from pushing, and it generally would not take away the urge to push. However, it does keep her from adding the voluntary strength to a pushing effort.

Breathing for Birth

1. *Breathing the baby out* She is asked to breathe in deeply, then while exhaling gently push downward with abdominal muscles visualizing the baby moving down and out. It may help to grunt or vocalize while exhaling. Continue this pattern throughout the contraction.

2. *Pushing the baby out* During a contraction when the urge to push becomes irresistible, then she is asked to hold breath for five to seven seconds while pushing. She can then breathe deeply in and out again until the urge to push becomes strong. Repeat this throughout the contraction.

3. *'Purple' pushing* Holding the breath and pushing for as long as possible before coming up for air can cause a reduced oxygen supply to the fetus, and therefore is not recommended.

Chapter 10

Caesarean Section
An overview of caesarean section

The lower segment caesarean section (LSCS) is the surgical approach usually made transversely through lower uterine segment. It can be elective (planned) or emergency.

Procedure   This surgery is done using general anesthesia or regional (spinal / epidural). A caesarean can be planned in advance (elective section) or be performed at short notice particularly if there are complications or difficulty in labour (emergency section).

An elective caesarean section is performed one to two weeks before the baby's due date.

INDICATIONS FOR CAESAREAN SECTION

A caesarean may be the only safe option for mother and baby in some situations like

◎   The placenta lies so low in the uterus that it covers the exit to the birth canal (cervix). This is called *placenta previa*.

◎   The obstetrician finds out that baby's health is threatened due to lack of oxygen.

◎   There is vaginal bleeding and a natural delivery is not about to happen.

◎   The umbilical cord falls forwards and the baby cannot be delivered easily (a condition known as cord prolapse).

◎   It becomes clear during labour that the woman will be unable to deliver the baby herself.

In other situations a caesarean may be considered the safest option even though a vaginal birth is a possibility.

◎ If the baby is lying with its head upwards (breech baby). This position is shown in Fig. 10.1.

◎ If the mother is affected by high blood pressure or other illness.

◎ If the unborn baby is too small or too weak to survive a natural birth.

◎ If the mother has had a caesarean delivery before (although it is possible for a mother who's had a caesarean to have a vaginal delivery in a later pregnancy).

◎ If the amniotic fluid is just adequate.

Fetus in breech position

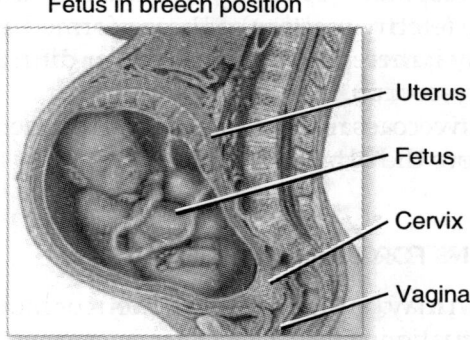

Fig.10.1 *Foetus in breech presentation*

In very rare cases, when the mother is so anxious about the delivery that a caesarean is considered.

If the surgical procedure is planned, then preoperative physiotherapy can be advised.

Aims

The Aims are:

a. To keep airways clear and maintain lung capacities.

b. To maintain mobility of the pregnant lady.

c. To take care of pain and keep pain levels low.
d. To keep the lady psychologically motivated

The operation is done with a team of doctors with the help of midwives and nurses. An incision of 20 cm long is given across the lower abdomen using spinal or epidural anesthesia (Fig. 10.2). The abdomen is opened up and baby is taken out carefully and finally sutures are given to seal the abdomen. This procedure, called the Caesarean section (Fig. 10.3), takes 20–30 minutes.

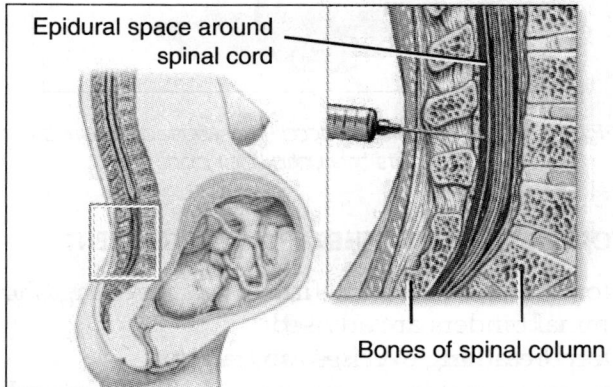

Epidural space around spinal cord

Bones of spinal column

Fig. 10.2 *Spinal/epidural anaesthesia*

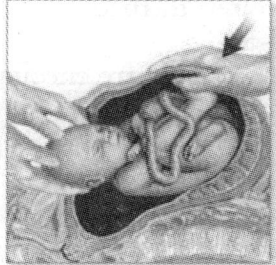

With both hands, the surgeon reaches into your uterus and lifts your baby's head as an assistant pushes down on your upper uterus to help guide your baby out

Fig. 10.3 *Caesarean section. The surgeon reaches into the uterus with both hands and lifts the baby's head while the assistant pushes down on the upper uterus to help guide the baby out*

After the completion of the surgery the cord is clamped and cut by the surgeon as shown in Fig. 10.4.

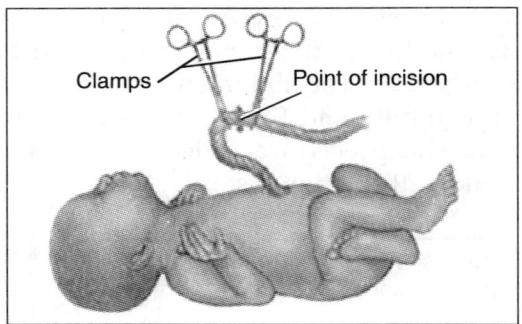

Fig. 10.4 *The umbilical cord: The surgeon clamps and cuts the umbilical cord*

POSTOPERATIVE PHYSIOTHERAPY MANAGEMENT

Comfortable clothes – like firm pants, cycling shorts and abdominal binders are advised.

1. Deep breathing exercises are taught.
2. Splinted coughing is encouraged with use of pillows on the incision site.
3. Ankle and toe pumps, ankle foot exercises are insisted to prevent DVT and aid circulation.
4. Encourage movements around the bed.
5. Begin quadriceps, glutei sets.
6. Pelvic rocks and straight leg raises are encouraged.

Management

1. TENS, hot-packs to relieve pain levels.
2. Correct seating techniques.
3. Avoid lifting heavy weights.
4. Sitz baths.
5. Use of coccyx wedge pillows.

Chapter 11
Postnatal Period

This is the period after the delivery of baby through the phase of labour. In this period, the lady is advised to undergo exercises, after she is comfortably adjusted with the baby and postdelivery conditions.

She is taught in her antenatal classes about some part of management of her postnatal challenges, baby care, which includes nappy changing, breast feeding, baby bathing and massage, etc. which she is reviewed again.

She is taught about diastasis recti and the importance of exercises. Pelvic training, Kegel's exercises, Aerobics, Hydrotherapy is also included in the session.

She is also treated for her postnatal pains, aches and discomforts, through therapeutic modalities as well as with the aid of exercises and assistive devices.

The benefits of postnatal exercises are follows.

- Speedier healing and recovery from the rigors of birth.
- Faster return to your prepregnancy shape and level of fitness.
- Increased energy to cope with the demands of new motherhood.
- Reduced stress and depression.

Tips

- Exercises should be strictly avoided for at least the first three days after the delivery.
- Avoid heavy lifting for a few weeks.
- Wear an appropriate bra that offers good support.

◎ Should not do any exercises that hurt the breasts.
◎ She may try to exercise after breastfeeding, rather than before when her breasts are full and heavy.
◎ Aim to exercise three or four days per week.
◎ If she feels breathless or light-headed while exercising, she should slow down or stop.
◎ If she experiences any changes in her postnatal vaginal flow (lochia), such as increased heaviness or changes in color, she should see her doctor as she may be exercising too strenuously.

EXERCISES IN POSTNATAL PERIOD

◎ Ankle pumps to aid circulation in lower limbs and prevent chances of DVT.
◎ Upper limb exercises –strengthening exercises of arms such as shoulders, elbows, hands etc., helping to carry the baby for long periods.
◎ Rectii abdominal strengthening (in line of diastasis recti)
   a. Curl-ups, curls-downs
   b. Obliques strengthening exercises.
   c. Exercises in different grades as the muscles get strengthen-to start with hands by sides in crook lying position, then arms crossed in front of chest, then hands behind head.
◎ Pelvic floor exercise/Kegel exercises
These exercises help to relieve pain by alternate repeated contractions and relaxations of the muscles. Their effects are as follows.
   a. To aid venous and lymphatic drainage.
   b. To help in removal of traumatic exudates.
   c. To stimulate the pain gate pathways in turn release of endogenous opiates to have pain relief.
      ◎ Stretching exercises lengthen the muscles (like hip flexors, piriformis, pectorals, calf) as they get shortened in response to skeletal changes during pregnancy. To stretch left piriformis: The lady is in

supine lying position with instructions to flex the hip, adduct and externally rotate with body weight lowering towards the right side.

Precautions

1. Not to push into extreme range of movement
2. Discourage ballistic bouncing
3. Discourage use of assistance as it reduces the control of safe stretch
   ◎ Relaxation techniques
   ◎ Posture care
   ◎ Baby care
   ◎ Counselling

Types of Aerobic Exercises

Recommended postnatal exercises include:
◎ Brisk walking
◎ Swimming
◎ Aqua-aerobics
◎ Low impact exercises

BABY CARE

1. Nappy Changing

While changing nappies, which is usually 8–12 times a day, the lady should handle herself with care.
◎ She should avoid bending her back often as shown in Fig. 11.1.
◎ It is done on her lap with her back supported.
◎ She changes nappy at the height of her waist and avoid stooping (Fig. 11.2) .
◎ Half kneeling is also preferred, as shown in Fig. 11.3.

2. Baby Bathing

◎ Use large bath tubs where mother can give bath to baby in standing (Fig. 11.4) or half- kneeling posture.

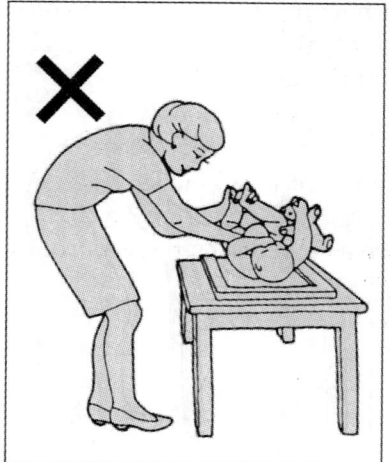

Fig. 11.1 *Nappy changing: Mother should not bend*

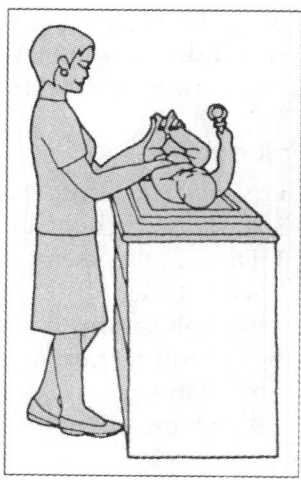

Fig. 11.2 *Nappy changing in standing position*

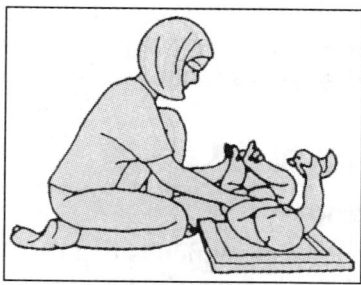

Fig.11.3 *Comfortable position in sitting posture*

◎ Strictly avoid buckets full of water as they put strain on her back.

◎ Keep the bathing accessories like towel and soaps or lotions close to the bathing area.

3. Breast Feeding

Breast feeding is a personal decision for the mother to make. The first step towards successful breast feeding is to make the decision before having a baby.

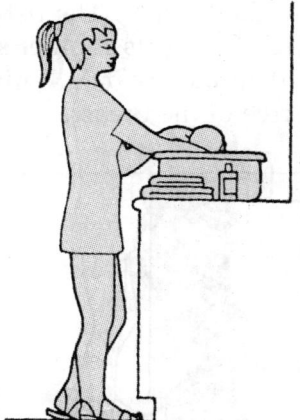

Fig.11.4 *Baby bathing using a bathtub*

Breast feeding can begin immediately after the baby is born. Immediately after birth the baby is often awake. It eagerly searches for the breast and wants to suckle. The baby can be helped by carefully supporting it under the soles of its feet so it can crawl or push itself up from the stomach and all the way to the breast. It will eagerly search for the breast and start suckling as soon as it is there. It is important that the breasts are stimulated as soon as possible, as the quantity of milk depends on how often the baby suckles.

Positioning During Breast Feed

The growing breast during 5 months of pregnancy needs attention of the 'would be mother' as breasts serve the food for the baby.

1. The lady is taught 'to always' wear her inner wear *(brassieres).*
2. She should wear the appropriate size of brassieres, preferably with the straps open in front for comfortable feeding (Fig. 11.5).
3. The mother should get as comfortable as possible so that the back and arms are supported. Then the baby should

be laid close to the mother. The baby should be lying with its stomach facing its mother's stomach with its head bent a little backwards. This way its nose is automatically free of the breast.

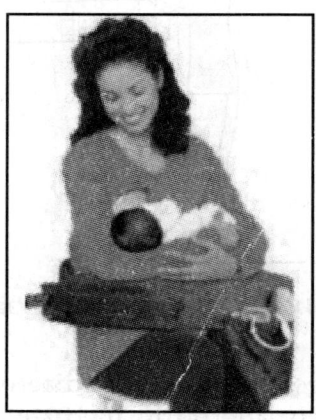

Fig. 11.5 *Breast feeding*

4. If sitting on a chair, mother sits in the rear of the seat, her back supported with a cushion, and a cushion or pillow kept in the lap to raise the head of baby, close to breast with a foot stool, under her feet, keeping knees 90 degrees flexed (Fig. 11.6).
5. Side-lying position either right or left, baby close to breast, supported with a pillow underneath the baby (Fig. 11.7).
6. Half kneeling is preferred than kneeling as it is very painful for her back.
7. Avoid leaning backwards while breast feeding
8. Do practice thoracic extension and scapulae retraction twice a day.
9. Avoid the development of heavy sagging breasts.

Change the breast every 10 minutes to maintain the baby's interest and to get them to drink as much as possible. It helps in holding the baby a lot, stroke its entire body and massage

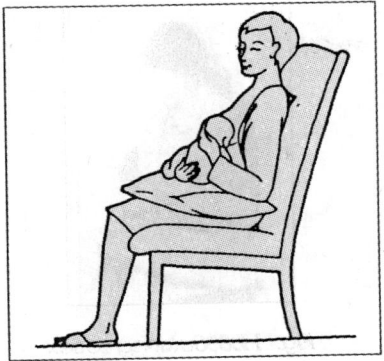

Fig.11.6 *Breast feeding: In relaxed sitting*

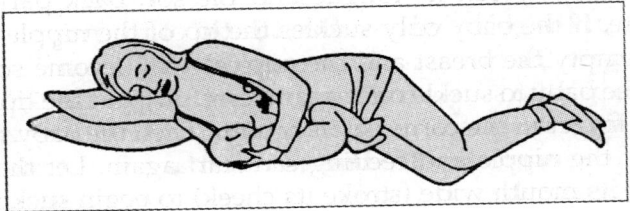

Fig. 11.7 *Breast feeding : In right side lying*

him or her gently. Caressing or talking to baby stimulates them to wake up.

Stimulation of Suckling Mechanism

Most babies are eager to suckle as soon as they feel the nipple against their cheek. If the baby is not reacting or is too sleepy, the suckle reflex can be stimulated by gently stroking the baby's cheek and lips with the fingertips, as seen in Fig. 11.8. The baby will then turn its head and search for the nipple with an open mouth. The lady should not stroke both cheeks as it will confuse the baby.

The whole nipple and its brown circle (areola) should get into the baby's mouth or the baby will not be able to create a

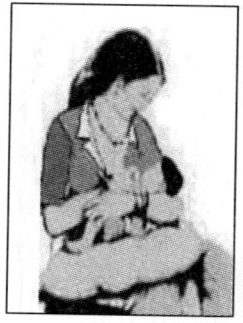

Fig. 11.8 *Sucking reflex*

vacuum between its tongue and the soft back part of its palate. If the baby only suckles the tip of the nipple it will not empty the breast and the nipples will become sore. To get the baby to suckle once again, carefully put the tip of the little finger in the corner of its mouth. Then the baby will let go of the nipple and feeding can start again. Let the baby open its mouth wide (stroke its cheek) to begin suckling.

WEANING FROM BREASTS

To get into the habit of taking the baby gently away from the breast, if the baby is pulled away in the middle of feeding, the mother's nipples will become sore quite quickly. Instead, put the tip of the little finger in the corner of the baby's mouth and he or she will automatically open his or her mouth. This will break the vacuum the baby creates in its mouth to suckle.

PRODUCTION OF MILK

When the mother feeds the baby, the suckling motion causes hormones to be released into the bloodstream from the pituitary gland in the brain. The hormones released are oxytocin and prolactin. Oxytocin causes the mammary glands in the mothers' breast to contract, so milk is released and flows to the baby. Many women experience this as a pulling sensation or a weight on their breasts when the baby begins suckling. The prolactin controls the amount of milk produced. The more the baby is fed, the more prolactin is released and the more milk produced.

Signs that Infant is Breast Fed

Good clues to be aware include the following:
◎ The baby wets six to eight nappies a day.
◎ The baby gains 100–200 g each week (around 400–800 g each month).
◎ The baby drinks as often as every two to three hours (around 8–12 times a day).
◎ The baby looks normal, has a nice colour and smooth skin, reacts normally, is strong and moves normally.

If the baby is sleepy and does not want to drink milk then he/she should be woken up and stimulated to drink every two hours, every day.

Chapter 12
The Puerperium and Postnatal Problems

THE PUERPERIUM

This is the final stage with a duration of 6–8 weeks postdelivery. The induction phase, i.e. the phase in which the woman's genital tract returns to the nonpregnant state. This follows, the third stage, in which the placenta and cord are expelled out.

Involution Phase

1. Reduction in size of uterus
   ◎ 1st day postpartum, it is above the umbilicus.
   ◎ 8th day postpartum, it is above midway between umbilicus and symphysis.
   ◎ 10th day postpartum, it comes back to its position that is behind symphysis, that is, in a span of 10 days from an abdominal organ, uterus turns back into a pelvic organ.
2. Laxed vagina which is painful on movement slowly takes its normal form.
3. Retraction of uterine muscle.

Problems of Puerperium

1. There was excess fluid retention during pregnancy which is released in this phase, by increasing the frequency of micturition.

2. This is often accompanied with pain on micturition and or stress incontinence.
3. Lochia: It is similar to heavy periods. As it is alkaline in nature, which is the favourable environment for the organisms, chances for infections are high.
4. A feeling of labour type pain in lower abdomen, which gets referred to lumbar region. This pain is explained as throbbing, cramping or aching by the lady.
5. Trauma to urethra, ligaments, cervix, perineal areas, episiotomy or use of forceps are some of the reasons for pain. This pain can be graded by McGill pain questionnaire.

POSTNATAL PROBLEMS

◎ Painful perineum
◎ Postpartum haemorrhage
◎ Diastasis rectii
◎ Post natal pain:
 • Backpain
 • Neckpain
 • Coccydynia
◎ Symphysis pubic pain
◎ Incontinence—bladder and bowel
◎ Sacroiliac joint dysfunction
◎ Carpal tunnel syndrome
◎ Postnatal depression
◎ Puerperal psychosis
◎ Problems due to nerve compression
◎ Brachial plexus pain
◎ Posterior tibial nerve compression
◎ Costal marginal pain
◎ Chondromalacia patellae

◎ Varicose veins

◎ Meralgia paresthetica

◎ Cramps

PAINFUL PERINEUM

This is the immediate happening after the delivery, and it includes problems like

   i. Bruising
   ii. Edema
  iii. Labial tears
  iv. Haematoma
   v. Infections
  vi. Haemorrhoids
 vii. Breakdown of sutures
viii. Vaginal haematoma

Laceration in perineum is divided into four degrees.

◎ *First degree:* Laceration confined in vaginal mucosa and skin of perineum

◎ *Second degree:* The laceration extends into perineal muscles.

◎ *Third degree:* This extends till the external anal sphincter muscles.

◎ *Fourth degree*: Deepest involving anal sphincter and anal mucosa.

Management

1. As pain is a dominant feature, cold therapy is easy to apply, fast – pain relieving agent. Warm baths, saline baths are also used. Cold therapy has an edge over the warm bath and tends to increase edema and sensitivity to pain. Ice packs are applied for 10–15 minutes at equal intervals between two-four hours for 3 days. Slowly as pain and bruising are reduced, ice is weaned off.

2. Ultrasonic therapy under water bag over painful region with dosage of 1 or 3 MHz in crook-lying position.
3. Elevate the foot end of bed.
4. Ankle and foot exercises to aid circulation in lower limbs.
5. Slowly pelvic floor exercises are started.

Posture Care

1. Cushion under buttocks while sitting.
2. Firm fitting underpants so that sanitary pad is in place, avoiding friction to painful perineum.
3. Correct defecation technique so that pain does not shoot-up.

POSTPARTUM HAEMORRHAGE (PPH)

This is loss of blood from genital tracts during and after delivery in excess of 560 ml with in first 24 hours. After this period, it is known as secondary PPH.

Causes

1. Usually it is uterine atoning. The uterus fails to contract and control the bleeding from placental site.
2. Birth canal trauma.
3. Retained placental tissue: There are some placental fragments remaining and uterus is not able to contract downwards.
4. Gravitational edema.
5. Puerperal infections. There are infections in genital tracts.

Secondary PPH

This occurs from 24 hours after delivery until the end of puerperium.

DIASTASIS RECTI

Diastasis or Divarication means a split between the two rectii abdominis muscles mostly seen in women with full term.

Measurements of gap varies from 2–3 cm wide and 12–15 cm long to a space measuring 12–20 cm in width and goes to whole length of rectii.

Women with a narrow pelvis, those who delivered large babies or who had a multiple birth (multiparae), are at risk of having a gross diastasis.

Test: The lady is in crook lying, physiotherapist places her hand width-ways below umbilicus and commands or instructs the lady to lift her head and reach with her hands towards her knees. If the diastasis is less than two fingers in width, abdominal exercises can be started. If the gap is greater, rotation and side flexion exercises should be postponed. These movements can increase the gapping because of shearing forces.

In some women "peaking" of abdomen is found which shows severe degree of diastasis.

The lumbosacral fascia, obliques group, transversus abdominis, become weak. There is loss of stable interrelationship between attachment and muscle fiber direction. Changes in angle of insertion influences the line of action which in turn reduces functional ability.

The changes in hormonal levels, mechanical stresses, ligamentous laxity causes the bulging of the muscles.

Re-education

1. The lady should be taught to palpate her own abdomen and feel the diastasis during her three trimesters.
2. Explain her about the action area of muscle and its role in the body, in simple words.
3. Make the woman aware of her abdomen in all positions.
4. After the theoretical understanding, practical demonstration about the diastasis, and prevention of diastases need to be done.

Exercises

1. Abdominal retraction should be repeated frequently.

2. Pelvic tilting (a dynamic exercise) should be taught in crook and side lying, sitting and standing.
3. Exercises can be made difficult by adding pelvic tilt with head and shoulder raising in crook lying.
4. To start with, to support head and upper trunk, several pillows can be used as a support.
5. Later, to improve abdominal strength, these pillows are removed and thereby, resistance of gravity and range of movement are increased.
6. Crook lying, mother crosses her hands over abdomen, fingers outside the lateral border of rectii, and then oppose, with head and shoulder raise.
7. *Peaking of rectii:* The separation of rectii exceeds 25 cm or more, i.e. the diastasis is quite wide, then the keeps her hands cross over the abdomen placing her fingers outside the lateral borders. She then raises her head and shoulders at the point of peaking, holds the position for 4–6 counts and then lowers slowly.
8. Avoid/delay side-flexion and rotational activities as shearing forces can increase the problem.
9. Single and double leg-sliding and curl-downs are safe.
10. The prime role of abdominal is to provide stability to spine, which occurs through isometric co-contraction. Therefore, transversus abdominis activation with co-contraction of pelvic floor is taught in modified four-point kneeling position, she is taught to practise this exercise in early postnatal period.
11. The exercise in prone kneel position is as follows. Towel roll is kept under the ankles, forearm resting on stool/chair. The physiotherapist places her hand on lower abdominal wall and gives the command to the patient to "breathe in, breathe out, slowly draw the abdomen towards the spine and away from hand".

    Hold the contraction for 10 seconds, while holding this contraction she is encouraged to draw the pelvic floor up.

Precaution: A full bladder can inhibit the contraction.

13. Later, when she masters 10 sec hold for 10 times, she can go to sitting with backward inclination. Place thumbs on ASIS and first finger on rib – for biofeedback of spinal alignment. She is commanded to extend the hip, maintaining co-contraction of pelvic floor and abdominals.

14. Tubi-grip (double-thickness), roll-on/pantie-girdle can be used as abdominal support (Fig. 12.1). Use of abdominal supports and corsets are used to give extra, safe support. They act as stimulators for active contraction of abdominals but she should not lean on the corset as it causes her laxed or less toned abdominals to deteriorate.

Commands are given to "Draw the belly in". After the pain is relieved and abdominals are strong, slowly corset can be weaned off.

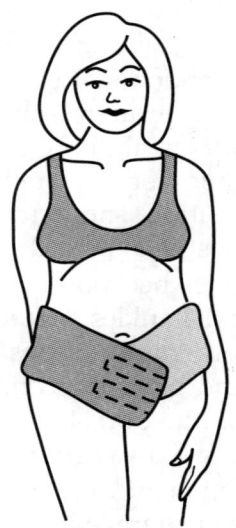

Fig. 12.1 *Lumbar belt*

PAIN IN POSTNATAL PERIOD

◎ Back pain
◎ Neck pain
◎ Coccyodynia

Neck Pain

It is a very common complain where either it is localized to one area or it includes neck, upper back and rarely even the tingling/radiating pain in the arm.

Causes

a. Prolonged bending to feed the child.
b. Adopting bad sleeping postures.
c. Advent of early degenerative changes in the cervical vertebrae.

Treatment

1. The lady is advised to do gentle neck exercises, which involves moving neck in the following different directions.
   a. *Flexion:* Forward bending of neck-touch the chin to the chest.
   b. *Extension:* Backward bending of neck, try to see the ceiling.
   c. *Side-flexion:* Touch the ear to the shoulder.
2. The lady should do these exercises every two hours.
3. The lady should avoid jerky movements.
4. She should use a soft thin pillow or a cervical butterfly pillow.
5. Maintain an erect and tall posture.
6. Use a chair with high back-rest.
7. While feeding, keep the baby close to the chest.

Coccydynia

Usually, the lady complains of pain in tail bone area after long hours of sitting or during defecation and coughing.

Causes

1. Stretching or rupture of ligaments during labour, accompanied with or without posterior displacement of coccyx.
2. Soft tissue damage (neuritis of coccygeal plexus).
3. Fracture of ankylosed sacrococcygeal segment.

Therefore, to get in control
1. The lady is advised to shift weight from one buttock to other.
2. Use of coccyx wedge pillows gives no strain for coccyx.
3. The lady is advised to sit tall and erect, allowing the weight transmission through ischial tuberosity.
4. Use of lumbar roll reduces the strain on coccyx.
5. Side sitting and side lying positions Are advised as these are pressure-relieving positions for coccyx.
6. Pelvic floor exercises, leg lift exercises are prescribed.
7. A detailed advice on posture care is given.
8. Avoid forward flexion movement.
9. Good fluid intake with plenty of roughage in diet is advised as it prevents constipation to a great extent.

SYMPHYSIS PUBIS PAIN

Symphysis Pubis Dysfunction/Diastasis of Symphysis Pubis in Pregnancy

Many pregnant women have the complaint of pubic pain during their pregnancy usually at the end of first trimester and some suffer even postnatal. Other names of DSP are public shear, symphyseal separation, pubic symphysis separation, separated symphysis, pelvic girdle relaxation of pregnancy, or pelvic joint syndrome.

Symphysis pubis dysfunction states that there is abnormally wide gap between the pubic bones at the symphysis pubis joint.

The gap in a nonpregnant woman is around 4–5 mm. During pregnancy, there is at least 2–3 mm increase in the gap due to influence of relaxin and the growing fetus. There is a decrease in this extragapping within three to five months postpregnancy. Abnormal gap of 1 cm or more is called 'separation of symphysis pubis'.

Symphysis pubis plays a vital role in holding the pelvis steady during any activity, and in any position which involves the legs. Even the sacroiliac joints are equally affected by the influence of pregnancy, which in turn increases the stress on symphysis pubis.

Causes

1. Usually as a result of increase in hormones during pregnancy.
2. If the woman had preexisting elevation in her hormonal levels (before pregnancy), there is an abnormal rise in pregnancy hormones resulting in excessive relaxation of ligaments, especially in pelvis.
3. Lots of children / had large babies.
4. Preexisting pathology in the joint.
5. Preexisting back pain / pelvic pain.
6. Trauma.
   a. Broken pelvis
   b. Obstetric trauma which have damaged the pelvic girdle area (mishandling during birth of the baby).
7. Hypomobile ladies.
8. Misalignment of the pelvis often associated with malposition of the baby like breach or occiput posterior

Symptoms

1. Pain
   Pubic pain
   Low back pain in sacroiliac area
   Sciatic pain involvement
   Occasionally, knee pain which may be radiating from pelvic area
2. Tenderness
3. Patient has difficulty in
   a. Rolling in bed

b. Coming up in the bed
c. Walking, especially after sleep
d. Sitting down or getting up
e. Bending, putting on clothes
f. Lifting heavy objects
g. Standing on one foot

Coping with Pubic Symphysis Pain

If the causative factor is misalignment in the joint, chronic SPD pain can be resolved by realigning the pelvic girdle and soft tissues. Most women have at least some residual pubic and low back pain stick around during pregnancy and the early postpartum weeks because of hormonal changes.

Tips

◎ Use a pillow between the legs when sleeping.
◎ Use a thin pillow or towel roll under tummy when sleeping.
◎ Keep the legs and hips as parallel as possible when turning in bed.
◎ Deep water aerobics or deep water running may be helpful as well.
◎ Keep the legs close together and move symmetrically.
◎ When standing, stand symmetrically, with the weight evenly distributed through both legs.
◎ Sit down to get dressed, especially when putting on underwear or pants.
◎ Avoid 'straddle' movements.
◎ Swing the legs together as a unit when getting in and out of cars.
◎ An ice pack may feel soothing and help reduce inflammation in the pubic area.
◎ Move slowly and without sudden movements.
◎ Really severe cases may need crutches, although this should be used only as a last resort.
◎ Sciatica may be helped by stretching the hamstring muscles with a stirrup around the foot.

◎ Back pain can often be helped by resting backwards over a large gymnastic or birth ball.
◎ Pelvic binders or maternity support belts are helpful for pelvic pain.

Inactivity may lead to atrophy and regular exercises is helpful in prevention of many common pregnancy problems. In severe cases, where a few minutes of activity is very uncomfortable, then bed-rest is opted.

URINARY INCONTINENCE

It is defined as the involuntary loss of urine. Women suffer from this condition four times more than men.
The possible causes could be as follows.

1. Trauma during childbirth.
2. Loss of estrogen from menopause.
3. Genetic reasons.
4. Stress, tension or anxiety.

Urine outflow is controlled by the contraction of detrusor and other bladder muscles along with sphincters opening and closing with pressure gradient. This is shown in Fig. 12.2.

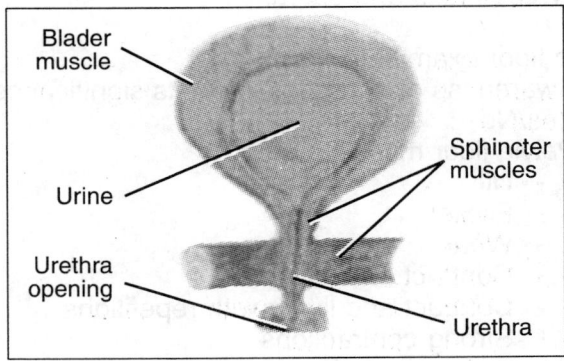

Fig. 12.2 Urine control mechanism

INCONTINENCE ASSESSMENT FORM

Name :

Age :

Occupation :

Subjective complaints (in patient's own words) :
Aggravating factors:
Coughing /sneezing/lifting weights:

Medical/surgical history

Obstetrics and gynaecological history :
◎ Number of deliveries
◎ Type of deliveries — normal/cesarean
◎ Any miscarriages/abortion — if yes, give details
◎ Any contraceptive methods — give details

Bladder functions
◎ Frequency of using the toilet
◎ Urgency
◎ Nocturia
◎ Type of incontinence
◎ Onset of incontinence
◎ Number of panties/pads changed per day (pad test)
◎ Water intake and output

Pelvic floor examination
◎ Awareness of pelvic floor and its significance :
Yes/No
◎ Pelvic floor muscle strength :
0 - Nil
1 - Flicker
2 - Weak
3 - Contract and lifting
4 - Contract and lifting with repetitions
5 - Strong contractions
◎ Any other complains

Management
- ◎ Short-term goals
- ◎ Long-term goals
- ◎ General outline of incontinence management :
  1. Kegel exercises
  2. Mid-flow urine exercises
  3. Bladder retraining
  4. Electrical stimulation
  5. Biofeedback to assist in retaining pelvic floor muscles
  6. Home advice

To start the Kegel exercises :
- ◎ The lady is positioned in supine lying with hip and knees flexed. Ask the lady to keep her hand on pubic hairline area to appreciate contraction.
- ◎ She will contract her pelvic floor by lifting up and back.
- ◎ The exercises are taught with a very simple analogy.
- ◎ The lady imagines she is on ground floor, to go up to fifth floor she should take her pelvic floor area up and hold it for five counts and then slowly relax, while she considers herself coming down from fifth floor to the ground level.

Once the exercises are mastered, the lady is taught to practise these in different positions:
1. Supine lying with hips and knees flexed
2. Prone kneeling/on all fours
3. Sitting on chair with arms across the body
4. Forward lean standing

Devices like perinometer and vaginal cones are used as modes of resisted exercises to pelvic floor muscles.

Perinometer
It is a pneumatic device which can be used to practise pelvic floor exercises. A hygienic, sterilized, compressible, air-filled rubber segment (sensor) is inserted into the vagina attached by a rubber tubing to a manometer.

When lady contracts, this pneumatic sensor compresses, increasing the reading on dial giving a visual clue to the lady to perform her exercise regimen.

Vaginal Cones

They are used for effective strengthening of pelvic floor muscles. In positions like half-lying, semi-sqatting/standing with one leg on a stool. Cones are inserted so that they can stand vertically above the level of pelvic floor. The lady is then asked to squeeze the cone, thereby strengthening her weak muscle group. She is advised to walk for 15 minutes with the vaginal cones for strengthening the muscles.

Electrical stimulation to the pelvic floor muscles helps in reeducating the muscle groups and strengthening too. In this, the lady lies in sideline position with pillows between her legs. The large pad electrode is placed on the lumbosacral area and the vaginal electrode is inserted in vagina.

Faradic currents with surges with audio visual clues are provided for effective reeducation of pelvic floor muscles. This is done for a duration of 15 to 20 minutes.

Interferential Therapy (IFT)

It is transcutaneous application of alternating medium frequency electrical currents, amplitude modulated at low frequency for therapeutic purposes.

The process of amplitude modulation is achieved by mixing two out of phase medium frequency currents. Individual currents interfere with each other where they meet and set up a new wave form. Due to wave interference, the current amplitude sum algebraically.

The aim of IFT in treating stress incontinence is to increase the efficiency of sphincter muscles by stimulating the unstriped muscle with low frequency impulses to which it is sensitive and also by influencing the autonomic supply.

Position opted is stride sitting or crook stride lying.

Two electrodes are placed on the lower abdomen above the outer half of the inguinal ligament part of inner aspect of thigh, near the origin of adductors. The crossing point is at the urethral sphincter.

Carrier frequency of 2000 Hz is used
Sweep of 0–100 Hz can be opted.
10–50 Hz helps in stimulating the voluntary muscles of pelvic floor.

First treatment session is given for 8 minutes and is increased by 1 minute for each attendance up to 15 minutes.

Twice or thrice a week the treatment should be continued and adequate time is provided for the muscle to get trained.

A course of twelve treatments should be given.

Chronic, senile cases may need a second course of treatment.

Note:
◎ Avoid constipation
◎ Keep weight in control
◎ Avoid lifting heavy weights
◎ When the lady has mastered her pelvic floor contraction, she should contract them as a safeguard be-fore and during activities like lifting, coughing, sneezing, etc. which could lead to leakage of urine.

Types of Incontinence

1. Urge incontinence
2. Stress incontinence
3. Overflow incontinence
4. Reflex incontinence
5. Giggle incontinence

Urge Incontinence/Overactive Bladder

This is involuntary loss of urine with strong desire to void. This is of two types: sensory and motor.

Sensory Urgency

This is due to infection or stones or cystitis. In this condition the bladder fills easily but unwanted detrusor contractions are produced, either spontaneously or in response to activity.

Treatment
1. Pelvic floor exercises and bladder retraining.
2. Remove the infection or stones.

Motor Urgency

In this condition, the unstable detrusor is the cause. There is involuntary detrusor contraction either spontaneously or during activities like walking or coughing.

Treatment

1. Strong repeated pelvic floor contractions to suppress overactive detrusor action.
2. Bladder retraining.

Patients with urge incontinence are rehabilitated via pelvic floor exercises, interferential therapy for the pelvic floor muscles, and are taught how to control urgency, frequency and urine loss with urge suppression techniques and behavioral intervention.

Stress Incontinence

This is caused due to overweight in pregnancy which increases intra-abdominal pressure or after delivery in women or obese men.

During pregnancy, the growing uterus pushes the bladder down, therefore urine loss is felt as a dribble especially during cough or sneeze or any exertional activity.

After delivery, there is common complain of involuntary loss of urine in the absence of strong detrusor contraction or incompetent urethral closure mechanism. This is *genuine stress incontinence.*

Causes

a. Prolapse of bladder and urethra due to damage of supporting structures, i.e. muscles or nerves supplying sphincter or levator ani (during surgery/child birth) with uterine descent.
b. Fatigue or stretching from overuse repeated coughing,
c. Straining at stool due to constipation, lifting heavy weights or obesity.
d. Loss of pinchcock effect of intra-abdominal pressure

e. Atrophy associated with low levels of estrogen and aging or under-use.

Treatment

a. Pelvic floor therapy.
b. Four polar interferential therapy using adhesive sterile electrode.
c. IFT using sterile vaginal electrode stimulating the pelvic group.
d. EMG Biofeedback is the advanced method for strengthening and endurance training.
e. Personal hygiene by changing clean dried panties or using disposable ones.
f. Maintaining intake of water and at the same time the output / or the urine loss in a chart.

Strengthening Program

The lady should do pelvic floor contractions as taught via holding the pelvic structures up for maximum 8–12 contractions and sustain them for 5–6 seconds each. Do this series 3–4 times in a day and 3–4 days in a week.

Endurance Program

The lady should do pelvic floor contractions as taught via holding the pelvic structures as long as possible in sitting or lying. Then take rest for 5–7 seconds. Repeat this hold and rest for 3 times. This completes one set. Similarly, perform this set for four times, i.e. a set of 4. Continue working in sets of 4 for 10–20 minutes, preferably in mornings. The time of hold should be increased as the endurance improves.

Overflow Incontinence

Involuntary loss of urine due to overdistension of bladder. The urine gets stored in bladder but has difficulty in escaping.

Causes

1. Diabetic neuropathy: Impaired nerve supply to detrusor.
2. Obstructive urethra.
3. Overstretched detrusor.
4. Cauda equina lesions
5. Infections or fibrosis.

Treatment

1. Clear the fibrosis.
2. Diet and bowel training.
3. Intermittent self-catheterization.

Reflex Incontinence

Loss of urine due to overactivity of detrusor or involuntary urethral relaxation in the absence of sensory desire to void or due to neurological impairment.

Treatment

Bladder retraining.

Giggle Incontinence

This is seen during puberty, especially in young girls.

SACROILIAC JOINT DYSFUNCTION

Laxity of the joint allows repetitive movement at the sacroiliac joints to cause pain. This can be unilateral or bilateral. If it is unilateral, it will eventually lead to stress on the opposite side. Abnormal movement of the ileum with sacrum affects the position of the acetabulum. Bad postures during pregnancy period increases the chance of sacroiliac strain. Usually this shapes up in posterior pelvic stabbing, deep low back pain.

Management

1. The lady is made aware of her problem and its ways of solution.

2. The side lying position with pillows between the legs is the most comfortable position.
3. The use of orthotic devices like belts or corsets reduces the posterior pelvic back during activities.
4. Positional traction techniques are demonstrated and are taught to practise even at home. These techniques allow the sacroiliac joint gapping to relieve compression.
5. Lying supine, the affected leg is crossed over the sound leg to the maximum possible range where the sacroiliac joint is put under positional traction. She maintains this position for about 20–30 min twice a day.
6. Therapist controlled traction – Lying supine where the hands holding the sides of the bed the physiotherapist holding the affected leg above ankle joint, exerts a sustained longitudinal traction. This is practised bilaterally. This technique helps in relieving the compressive forces at the painful joint.

CARPAL TUNNEL SYNDROME

Compression of the structures of the wrist long flexor tendons in the confined space of the hand carpal tunnel which may or may not be accompanied with squeezing of the nerve which can lead to loss of sensation in the thumb zone and index and middle finger along with weakness of hand muscles.

The lady complains of pain in the wrist, which increases with repetitive activities like brushing, chopping, vegetables, etc.

Physiotherapy Management

As discussed before, the physiotherapy management is as follows.
1. Resting hand splints.
2. Strengthening exercise for the upper limb.
3. Specific gripping exercises.
4. Hand care.
5. Ultrasonic therapy at the painful wrist.

POSTNATAL DEPRESSION

Depression is a mental illness and when it occurs in the weeks or months after birth it is called postnatal depression.

◎ Around 10 to 15 per cent of all women develop some form of postnatal depression lasting more than two weeks.

◎ More than half of these women develop severe depression where medical treatment is considered necessary.

◎ Most serious depressions are apparent in the first month after childbirth, but they can also arise later.

◎ Without the right treatment, postnatal depression can last months.

The first few days, weeks and months after giving birth is a period of physical and psychological stress for both the new mother and father. The mother feels period of sadness or moodiness a couple of days after giving birth. This is both healthy and natural.

Sitting or lying with the newborn baby in the parent's arms is probably one of the happiest moments in the life of any man or woman. It is such a relief after so many months of waiting. The hardships of the pregnancy and the pain of delivery are forgotten for a while as a parent cuddles the tiny new arrival and feels a sense of tranquility. But most women will experience a period when they feel insecure, vulnerable, sad or anxious. The enormous responsibility of suddenly having a new baby to care for can make a new mother feel afraid and inadequate. Mood swings are common. It is possible to feel elated one moment and tearful, tired or irritable the next. This can be frightening too, not knowing what is happening or why the feelings are rising.

On the fourth day after the baby is born, mothers find themselves crying for no particular reason. This can happen at any time within the first week after the birth and usually passes in a day or two as long as the mother has had a chance to rest and is ready for her new world. Factors contributing to postnatal depression are as follows.

◎ Psychological and social factors such as the demands, obligations and responsibilities of being a mother.

◎ Family factors are also important, including the relationship a mother has with the child's father, and the support she receives from other people.

◎ Biological factors may also play a role including the hormonal changes that occur following the childbirth.

PUERPERAL PSYCHOSIS

Puerperal psychosis is a severe mental illness that occurs in about 1 in 500 deliveries. Sufferers may have a family history of psychotic illness, or have had a psychotic illness themselves in the past. In most cases, the onset is in the first two weeks after childbirth. The symptoms are usually an acute state of confusion, fluctuating mood, disordered thinking and behaviour and 'psychotic' symptoms of hallucinations and delusions. These delusions often take the form of irrational preoccupations concerning the newborn baby. In certain cases the baby may be at risk due to the mother's illness and a medical assessment is essential.

Treatment for puerperal psychosis is usually in the form of medication (usually antipsychotic and/or antidepressant medicines). Occasionally, electroconvulsive therapy (ECT) may be used.

PROBLEMS DUE TO NERVE COMPRESSION

The fluid retention during last phase of pregnancy creates the risk of compression of nerves in arms and legs.

Posterior Tibial Nerve Compression

Ankle edema can compress posterior tibial nerve as it passes behind the medial malleolus. This leads to paraesthesia of sole of foot and plantar aspect of toes.

Management

1. Ice-packs
2. Ankle and foot exercises
3. Leg elevation

BRACHIAL PLEXUS PAIN

Pain and paresthesia in shoulder and arm are the complains due to postural changes or structural anomalies like cervical rib, which shows symptoms due to the excess fluid in brachial region.

Management

1. Elevation of arm
2. Active exercises of upper limb
3. Strengthening exercises of shoulder and arm

COSTAL MARGINAL PAIN (RIB-CAGE PAIN)

Unilateral thoracic back pain along with the pain in anterior margin of lower ribs. This is due to growing uterus which ascends up in abdomen, forcing rib-cage to move outwards resulting in stretching of softened intercostal tissues. This is unilateral pain, radiating around the chest which may refer to lateral abdominal wall.

Management

'Rib-lifting technique' with heating pads is employed to relieve pain.

CHONDROMALACIA PATELLAE

"Chondromalacia" means softening of cartilaginous surfaces. The softening of cartilaginous surface of patella of knee in pregnancy is due to ligamentous laxity, prolonged stress of more body weight, wide pelvis and femoral torsion. In this condition, quadriceps or Q angle is increased.

Precipitating Factors
- Squatting activities
- Overweight: The pregnant lady puts on 20 kg more than her normal bodyweight.
- Activities in Kneeling position.

Management
- Ice packs – 2 to 3 times a day.
- Isometric exercises for quadriceps.
- Strengthening exercises for quadriceps.

VARICOSE VEINS

These are painful tortuous knotted veins

Causes
- Changes in the maternal blood circulation.
- Changes due to progesterone on smooth muscles or veins.

These give hypotonia with raised intra-abdominal pressure.

Precautions and Exercises
- Always elevate the legs while lying or sitting.
- Avoid sitting crossed legs.
- Always practise vigorous ankle pumps to aid circulation.
- Use compression stockings as they reduce edema by helping in venous return.

CRAMPS

Cramps are a very annoying problem faced by the lady postnatally. Cramps are commonly seen in calves and feet. As discussed earlier, ankle pumps and warm baths are helpful in reducing the cramps.

Chapter 13

Exercises for Week 6 and After

About six weeks after the baby's birth, the lady can do following activities to the beginning set of exercises. With a pair of 1.5- to 2.5-kg dumbbells, she can resume her arm-strengthening program at home. Later on she can add repetitions, sets of repetitions, and/or weights.

To begin the workout with a warm-up Start with the five minutes of marching, then add some shoulder rolls and shrugs, some knee bends and arm swinging, followed by regular stretches. Hold each stretch for eight to 10 seconds.

◎ Leg slide
◎ Leg fly
◎ Seated row
◎ Rear dumbbell fly
◎ Head and shoulder raises
◎ More advanced exercises
◎ Diagonal abdominal curl-ups

LEG SLIDE

1. The lady is in crook lying position with back on the floor and knees bent.
2. She tightens her abdominal muscles and presses the small of back against the floor as she breathes out.
3. Slides one leg away from her body slowly, using her abdominal muscles to keep back flat on the floor.

4. Then she moves the other leg, and eventually, slides both the legs together.

5. When the back starts to arch, she brings the legs back to the start position — keeping abdominal muscles pulled in. This is repeated eight to ten times.

LEG FLY

The lady lies on her side, where the lower leg is bent at hip and knee. The leg above is lifted up in the air and held for a count of 5 and then the she slowly brings it back (Fig. 13.1).

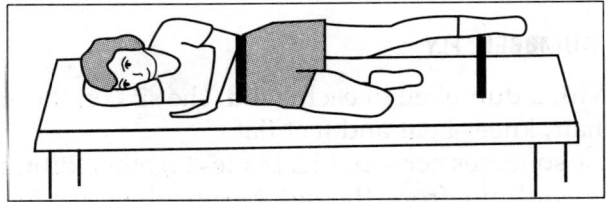

Fig. 13.1 *Abduction of hip*

WALL SLIDES

The lady slides on the wall where her back is maintained erect (Fig. 13.2).

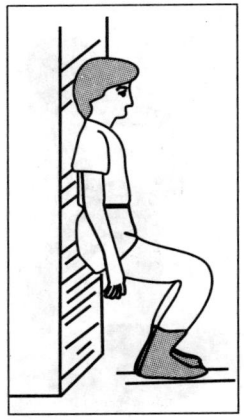

Fig. 13.2 *Wall slides*

SEATED ROW

◎ She sits on the edge of a chair, knees bent and feet flat on the floor, with a dumbbell on either side of her feet.

◎ Bend forward, bringing chest close to the thighs with back flat.

◎ Holding one dumbbell in each hand, let her arms hang straight down, palms facing each other.

◎ She lifts her elbows up, bringing them up towards the shoulders so that hands are level with knees. Lower the dumbbells to the floor and repeat eight to ten times.

REAR DUMBBELL FLY

◎ With a dumbbell in each hand, she sits on the edge of a chair, knees bent and feet flat.

◎ She squeezes her shoulder blades together, lifting elbows up and out from the sides until they are level with shoulders.

◎ Return the arms to starting position. Repeat eight to ten times.

This exercise can be performed even in standing position as a progression movement (Fig. 13.3).

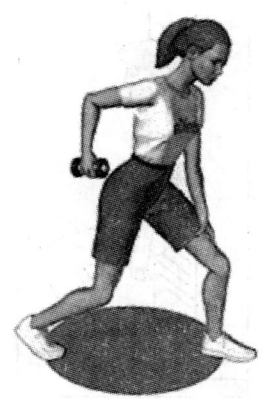

Fig. 13.3 *Dumbbell exercise*

WEIGHT CUFF LIFTS

◎ The lady is in prone-lying position at the edge of the bed.
◎ She lifts her left arm with the weight cuff tied above the wrist as seen in Fig. 13.4.

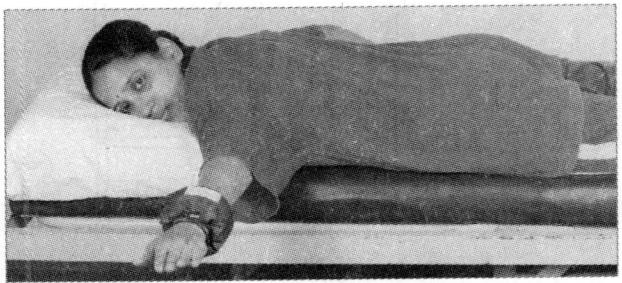

Fig. 13.4 *Triceps strengthening*

Note: The lady should remember to breathe normally and keep her abdominal muscles pulled in as she lifts. Exercises should not cause any pain in joints as joints are still affected by the hormonal changes of pregnancy. Weights should be reduced, if she experiences any discomfort.

THERABAND PULLS

◎ The lady sits on a stool with her neck and back straight with a theraband tied on a pole by the side (Fig. 13.5).
◎ She pulls the theraband with her hand away from her body and holds it there for a count of 5 and brings it back.
◎ She repeats with both the hands.

SPINE STRENGTHENING

◎ The lady lies prone (on her stomach) and with hands clasped behind, lifts her upper back (Fig. 13.6).

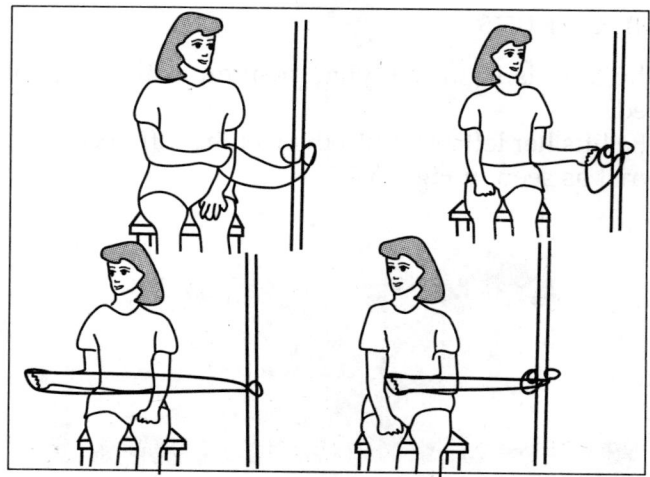

Fig. 13.5 *Theraband exercises*

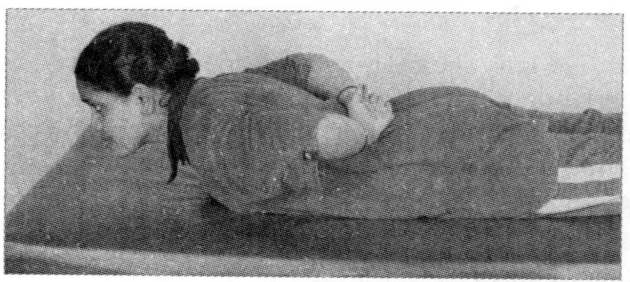

Fig. 13.6 *Upper back strengthening*

◎ The lady lies prone with weight cuff tied on her left leg lifted up in air without bending the knee (Fig. 13.7).

HEAD AND SHOULDER RAISES

More Advanced Exercises

After six-week check and provided the gap between the abdominal muscles is not more than two finger-widths apart (the "rec check"), she can progress with abdominal exercises.

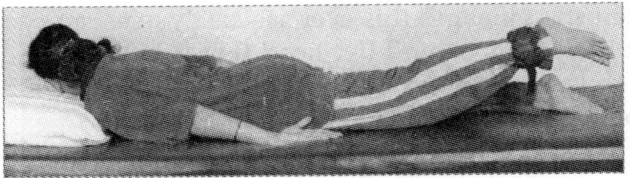

Fig. 13.7 *Hip and spinal extensors strengthening*

The following exercise is started only when she can perform abdominals with her hands by the body side without overtiring herself.

◎ She lies on her back with knees bent, feet flat on the floor, and arms crossed across her chest (Fig.13.8).

◎ Breathe in and as breathing out, pull in abdominal muscles, and lift head and shoulders off the floor.

◎ Make sure that she will keep her chin at the same angle to chest throughout the whole lift. Do not allow head to drop back and do not pull chin tightly down onto the chest.

◎ She lifts up herself as high as she feels comfortable and then lowers again. If she feels that abdominal muscles are bulging initially, then advice her not to lift high but try to control the abdomen and keep it as flat as possible while she lifts her head and shoulders.

◎ Repeat the sequence to 10 times.

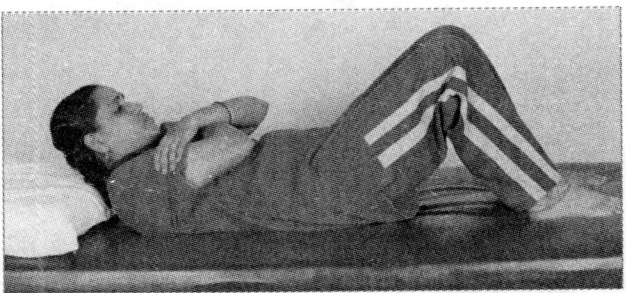

Fig. 13.8 *Hands across chest*

When she manages this exercise easily, she can progress to put her hands behind her head (Fig. 13.9). This requires more abdominal work and thus a stronger exercise. It can be too strainful if she progresses to it too soon.

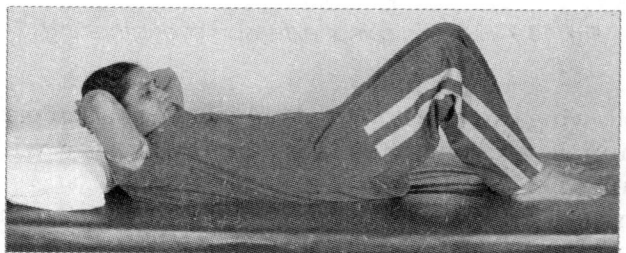

Fig. 13.9 *Hands behind head*

DIAGONAL ABDOMINAL CURL-UPS

It is most important not to progress to diagonal exercises until the gap between the abdominal muscles has healed and is two finger-widths apart or less — see the "rec check".

◎ Crook lying: She lies on her back with knees bent, feet flat on the floor, right hand on abdomen and left hand on the floor by the side. This position is shown in Fig. 13.10).

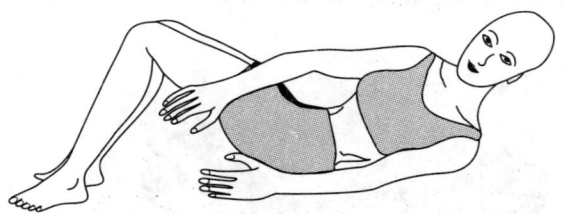

Fig. 13.10 *Oblique curl -ups*

◎ She breathes in and breathe out, pulls in abdominal muscles, and lifts head and shoulders off the floor, taking right hand towards the outside of her left knee.

◎ She takes care to keep chin at the same angle to chest throughout the whole lift and does not allow the head to drop back and does not pull chin tightly down onto the chest.

◎ She lift up only as high as comfortable and then lowers again. If there is a feel of abdominal muscles bulging initially, then does not lift so high but tries to control the abdomen and keep it as flat as possible while lifting head and shoulders.

◎ Repeats the exercise eight to 10 times, then changes hands and repeats on the opposite side.

BACK CARE

Tips and Toes

Instructions for the lady are as follows.

◎ Use appropriate baby lifting techniques (Fig 13.11).

◎ Always keep the back straight.

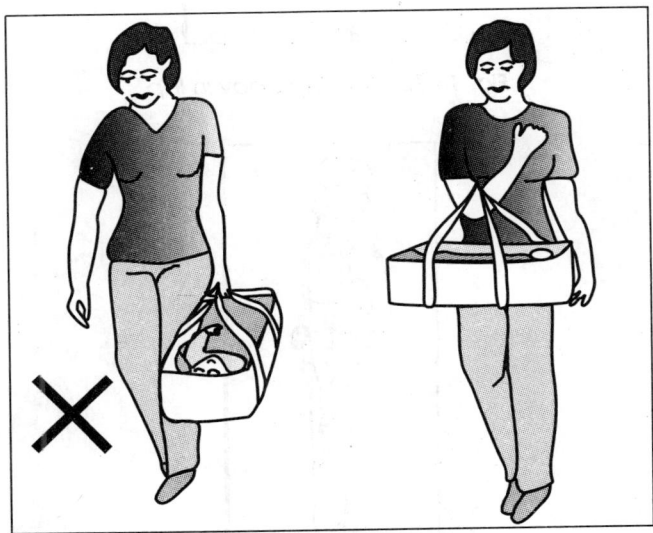

Fig. 13.11 *Baby lifting technique*

- Always hold the heavy weights or baby close to the body (Figs 13.12 and 13.13).
- Always divide the weights equally and carry in either hand.
- Always prefer pushing to pulling as it is energy saving (Fig. 13.14).
- Always keep the baby close to the breasts for baby feed.
- Prefer bending on hips and knees than with back.
- Avoid deep-knee bends / full squatting.
- Avoid extreme stretching or bouncy movements.

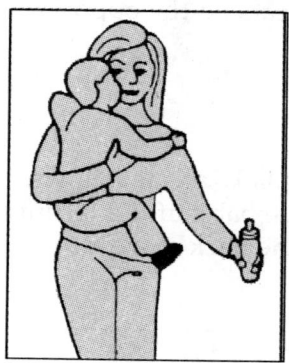

Fig. 13.12 *Carrying baby in lap*

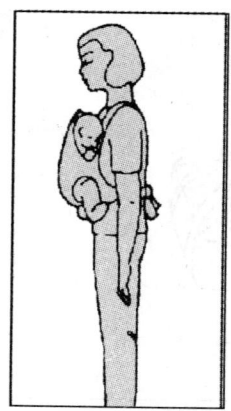

Fig. 13.13 *Carrying baby across the chest*

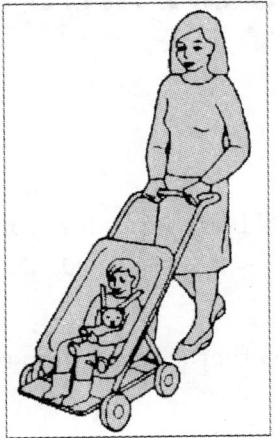

Fig. 13.14 *Pram baby handling*

Chapter 14

Fun Time

BODY TYPE

There are two MAIN body types for women:

◎ "Apple"
◎ "Pear"

There are also two other less common body types:

◎ "Celery" and
◎ "Cauliflower"

Basic Facts

1. You can have a heavy or a thin "apple" or "pear", but the weight will stay distributed around the areas specific to that body type.
2. An apple can't become a pear or visa versa. When pregnant, the apple is a "pregnant apple" and a pear is a "pregnant pear".
3. You can be a combination of two body types.

What is your Body Type?

1. The "**Apple**" carries weight around the middle. You have a strong, thickset skeletal frame with broad shoulders, a large rib cage, narrow hips and muscular limbs. Typically you can build muscle easily. You are fond of meat/protein.

2. The "**Pear**" on the other hand is "bottom" heavy. You have narrow shoulders, a relatively small waist, little lower tummy and larger hips and upper thighs. The buttocks are curved and rounded and the thighs extend outward laterally

and may touch or rub on the inside. Bread, chocolate and cheese (creams) are your favorites.

3. The "**Celery**" body is straight up and down. You typically like stimulants like coffee and cigarettes (hopefully not using either while pregnant!). The celery is thin and your weight gain in pregnancy is usually all tummy.

4. The "**Cauliflower**" body is round and puffy. You typically like salty food and put on weight evenly throughout your body. The "cauliflower" usually has problems with water retention

Bibliography

1. Guyton and Hall: *Textbook of Medical Physiology*, 10th edn, Saunders, 2001.
2. Carolyn Kisner and Colby: *Therapeutic Exercises*, 4th edn, Jaypee, 2000.
3. Clayton's *Electrotherapy Theory and Practice*, 9th edn, Forster and Palastanga, 1992.
4. *Physical Rehabilitation Assessment and Treatment*, 4th edn, Sullivan and Schmitz, 2001,.
5. *Women's Health: A Textbook for Physiotherapists*, Harcourt Brace, 1998.
6. *Physiotherapy in Obstetrics and Gynaecology*, Margaret Polden and Jill Mantle, 1994.
7. Cynthia Norkins: *Measurement of Joint Motion*.
8. Sembulingam: *Essentials of Medical Physiology*, 2nd edn.
9. Das, AK: *Medical Physiology*.
10. John Low and Ann Reed: *Electrotherapy Explained—Principles and Practice*, 3rd edn.
11. Michlovitz: *Thermal Agents in Rehabilitation*, 3rd edn.
12. Behrens and Michlovitz: *Physical Agents—Theory and Practice for the Physical Therapist Assistant*, 1996.
13. Wells and Frampton: *Pain Management by Physiotherapy*. 2ndedn, 1996.
14. John v. Basmajian: *Therapeutic Exercises*, 3rd edn, 1978.
15. Physical Therapy, *Journal of the American Physical Therapy Association*, **84**:2004.
16. Brenda Savage: *Interferential Therapy*, 1984; reprinted 1992 by Richard Clay Ltd.
17. Hamill, Knutzem: *Biomechanical Basis of Human Movement*, 2nd edn, 2003.
18. Davis and Harrison: *Hydrotherapy in Practice*.
19. Margaret Hollis and Phyl Fletcher-Cook: *Practical Exercise Therapy*, 4th edn.

Sites Referred

www.healthinsite.gov.au/topics/diet and pregnancy.
www.healthand yoga.com
www.nichd.gov/about/womenshealth/disorders of pregnancy
www.nichd.gov/about/womenshealth/breastfeeding.cfm
www.nichd.gov/about/womenshealth/prenatalcare.cfm
http://staging2/physiotherapy/anatomy.htm
http://staging2/physiotherapy/physiology.htm